The Medical Bill Survival Guide

Easy, Effective Strategies for People Experiencing Financial Hardship

Nicholas A. Newsad M.H.S.A.

ISBN 978-0-615-35283-1
ISBN 0615352839
LCCN - 2010924829

Cover Photo: © iStockPhoto, Jeffrey Smith
Cover Design by Andrew Brozyna, ajbdesign.com
Typeset by Jenni Wheeler

Printed in the United States of America

Blessed are the merciful,

for they will be shown mercy.

–Matthew 5:7

CONTENTS

INTRODUCTION

This book has wide appeal for those who need help with medical bills. To date I have not found a book that concisely describes the most effective strategies for managing medical costs and speaking to billers and collectors. I have assembled a straight-forward approach for doing exactly that. The most common problems that people struggle with in this respect are relatively simple to me because I've worked several years at the corporate level and on the front lines of a national healthcare management company and have a master's degree in hospital administration. The wide variety of medical bill problems makes it difficult to address every possible type of problem, so I've tried to focus on the most common issues. This book will benefit the following patients and patient families:

- Insured patients who are experiencing difficulty paying the deductibles, copays, and coinsurance.

- Uninsured patients who are unemployed or cannot afford health insurance.

- Patients and the families of patients who have survived a catastrophic medical episode like cancer, heart attack, or major surgery.

- Patients with chronic diseases requiring continuous, costly medical care like heart disease, COPD, or diabetes.

The very fact that you've selected this book tells me that you need help. You don't have to worry anymore. I've been there, on both sides of the phone, and it's going to be okay. The first thing I want to do is alleviate your anxiety by sharing a story about my first success as a patient advocate.

> *Carol was fifty years old and had not been to a gynecologist in twenty-five years. She had chronic pain for years and refused to see a physician. One day the pain was so unbearably excruciating that she was actually toying with the idea of going to an urgent care, but figured she might save a few dollars by first talking to her nurse sister-in-law Maggie. Maggie was appalled and immediately had Carol admitted to a hospital. This saved Carol's life, as she would have been dead within a few hours. Over the next two years, Carol would have multiple major surgeries, oncology treatments, and intensive care stays. She would lose over fifty pounds and all of her hair. She would have her colon detached, re-attached, and detached again forcing her to wear a colostomy bag for the rest of her life. She would also have a major relapse and remain comatose for over ten days after an emergency surgery.*

> *Though Carol was insured, she was stubbornly inclined to declare bankruptcy to wipe out the tens of thousands of dollars of deductibles, copays, and coinsurances she owed. I learned she was screening her calls so she wouldn't have to talk to billers and become angry and vulgar with those that did get through. She had ignored her financial problems in the same way she had ignored her disease and made virtually every wrong decision possible along the way.*

> *Despite ignoring her bills for the better part of a year, I spoke to over ten of Carol's providers about her situation over a six-week period and was able to eliminate the vast majority of her obligations. Her largest debtor, the hospital, ultimately waived 70% of her account balance because of my calls.*

I'm not in a secret club and there's no secret password. All of the things I said to Carol's billers are contained in this book. Carol was the quintessential procrastinator. She was and is the type of person who only goes to the dentist when the pain is so excruciating she cannot stand it. As a result, she often finds herself in anxious and frustrating positions. Dramatic emergencies that can't be ignored always happen to her because she puts off her small problems until they are monumental emergencies.

In my experience, anxiety and frustration can be cured 100% of the time by education. While this is a once-in-a-lifetime financial disaster that you may be experiencing for the first time, I've seen your problems many times from both sides of the desk and I'm going to show you how to take care of this.

You have to know the rules to play the game and I'm going to teach you the written and un-written rules of patient billing and collections. It's unfair that you be expected to understand what you are doing right from the beginning. When you really know what you're talking about, and you've read the many examples and anecdotes herein about other patients and their experiences, you'll be able to speak confidently and rationally to billers and get results.

Please note that this book will not be very helpful if you're exclusively trying to help an elderly parent pay for nursing home care. Long-term care nursing home bills are a completely different animal from acute medical care bills and chronic disease medical bills. If you need help with long-term care, I recommend you contact your state's ombudsman for aging or long-term care. These are full-time state employees that help people sign up for Medicaid with the specific intent to pay for nursing home care.

THINGS TO KNOW IF YOU HAVE INSURANCE

Even if you have health insurance, there is still a wide variety of problems that you may encounter. This chapter will explain the fundamental components of health insurance and describe six of the most common problems people experience related to coverage.

Health Insurance 101

Health insurance is a form of "risk pooling," which, basically, means that a large group of people agree to "share" the risk that a few of them may become sick by setting aside money (premiums) to pay for it when this happens.

Eighty-five percent of Americans are enrolled in some type of health insurance program. There are public insurance programs like federal Medicare for the elderly and disabled, state Medicaid for the poor, and SCHIP for children and pregnant women. There are also "private" or "commercial" insurance companies. These commercial companies sell insurance to employers who then provide it to employees as an employment benefit. Employers will pay the majority of the premium and the employee will pay a smaller part through payroll deductions. The five biggest commercial insurance companies in the U.S. are:

Rank	Company
1	UnitedHealth Group
2	WellPoint (Anthem)
3	Aetna
4	Humana
5	Cigna

One important thing to consider is whether your medical bill(s) stem from an auto accident or work accident. If your bills are related to an auto accident, your medical care is covered by the auto insurance company like GEICO, Allstate, or Amica. If you were injured in a work-related accident, your medical bills are covered by your state's Worker's Compensation Program. Your employer pays money into the state WC fund so that you're covered if you get hurt. This is important to note, because your employer-based health insurance will not want to pay if treatment is covered by another program.

Insurance companies do not pay 100% of your medical bills. You will still be responsible for an amount often referred to as the "patient responsibility." There are three types of patient responsibilities and they are called deductibles, copays, and coinsurance. Before I explain the difference, I want you to know why they exist. Studies have shown that when patients cost-share, they are likely to use less medical care. For example, patients who share the cost of their medical bills by paying 30% of their total medical bills use fewer medical services and go to the physician less than those patients that pay 20% of their medical bills. People who don't have to share the costs use the most medical care and go to the physician very frequently. Commonsense, right? If laundry detergent is more expensive, you're going to use slightly less per load and try to stretch your money further. If laundry detergent is free, you'll use much more, because there is no reason not to.

Deductible: This is a flat amount that you pay for medical care before insurance kicks in. Deductibles have been increasing significantly the past few years as insurance companies and employers try to shift more medical costs to employees. Whereas deductibles used to be $250-$500, they are now

$1,000-$5,000. For example, if you have a $1,000 deductible, you have to pay the first $1,000 of your bills and then insurance will kick in and start paying the rest of them.

Copay: This is a flat amount associated with certain types of care. Your employer chooses these copay amounts and they're spelled out in your benefit plan, as well as on your insurance card. For example, you might have a $25 copay for every visit with your family physician and a $50 copay with every visit with a specialist physician like a cardiologist or gynecologist.

Coinsurance: This is similar to copay, except it is a percentage, not a fixed amount. Your benefit plan will say where coinsurance is applied and where copays are applied. For example, you may have a 20% coinsurance for outpatient surgery. This means that the insurance company will pay 80% of the bill for the surgery and that you have to pay 20%.

If you have high patient responsibilities like a $3,000 deductible and coinsurances of 40% or higher, do not be upset at the insurance company. Your payments are high, because your employer chose an inexpensive health plan. I'll tell you what you can do about large patient responsibilities in a later chapter, but if you do find these costs to be high, I encourage you to let your employer's leadership know. They won't know unless you tell them. This is a major problem in the United States. Businesses are finding themselves in very competitive situations where they have to compete with companies in Europe and Asia that do not have to pay for employee health insurance.

Understanding in-network and out-of-network

You may have two sets of deductibles, copayments, and coinsurances if your health plan includes something called out-of-network (OON) benefits. To understand out-of-network benefits, you first have to know what in-network benefits are.

When your employer is trying to buy health insurance, the insurance company will offer them several different options called "health plans."

Different plans have different deductibles, copays, and coinsurances. Each plan is built around a unique set of providers that agree to provide medical care as part of the health plan. This includes physicians, hospitals, imaging centers, and other providers. If they agree to be in the plan, they are "in-network." In-network physicians and hospitals are the providers the insurance company wants you to see. The insurance company has checked to make sure that each one provides quality care and they have all agreed to a contract where the insurance company will pay them to take care of you.

Physicians and hospitals that are "out-of-network" are not in the health plan that your employer chose. Either the insurance company had an issue with the quality of the medical service or, more likely, they could not agree on the payment rates in a contract for paying the physician or hospital. If your benefit plan includes an out-of-network benefit, this means you're allowed to see a provider that is not in the health plan your employer chose, but the insurance company and your employer may try to dissuade you from seeing them by establishing higher deductibles and coinsurances for out-of-network physicians and hospitals. If your health plan doesn't include out-of-network benefits, then your insurance company won't pay for you to see those providers at all. If you see an OON physician and you have no OON benefit, you should tell them to treat you as if you have no insurance. I'll explain why later.

Why insurance may not pay and what to do about it

Every health insurance company has to have a physician to review claims. While people who work at these companies are very smart, they do not have licenses to make medical decisions, nor do they have the medical experience to understand specific problems. I once had the privilege of meeting the medical director of a major health insurance company. He spent several hours talking to me and several of my colleagues about why insurance companies sometimes do not pay and what to do about it. He talked about the six most common reasons claims are denied. I have listed these reasons below.

Incorrect policy number, enrollee number, or patient birth date

The claim that your physician or healthcare provider sent to the insurance company did not accurately identify who you are. This is the **number one reason for rejected or denied claims** and it is very common. This happened with several of Carol's providers. Check and double check to make sure the healthcare provider knows the name, policy number, enrollee number, and birth date of the policy holder and the patient, if they are not the same person. For example, Carol once mismatched her husband's enrollee number with her name. The insurance company claimed they had no such enrollee and the provider assumed she had no insurance. This was an easy fix once I talked to the biller at the hospital, but Carol had no idea what to look for.

Service not provided during enrollment period

Your employer buys health insurance every one to two years. Services that overlap these renewals periods are prone to errors. If your employer changes insurance companies, you have to be well aware of the effective dates and make sure your providers are well aware of the changes. If you lose your insurance and see a provider after it expires, you are an uninsured patient. This is not the end of the world. I will teach you what to do about this in the next chapter.

Service not a benefit in the enrollee's benefit plan

Your employer looks at many health plans and weighs the cost of the plan against the benefits and services included. Unfortunately, employers sometimes have to make tough decisions and cut certain benefits for the sake of others. What is even more unfortunate is that most employees, including me, never take the time to see what is included in their benefit plan until it is too late. If you get a notice from a healthcare provider or an EOB from your insurance company that states "service not a benefit in enrollee's plan" the first thing to do is check the benefit plan to make sure.

There are multiple places that this should have been caught before you received treatment. It is my opinion that providers should always "verify benefits" before performing any type of treatment. Verifying benefits minimally involves the business office getting online and checking to make sure that you are indeed covered and that you have benefits on your scheduled day of service. Some services additionally require pre-certification or pre-authorization by the insurance company. In this case, the provider should have acquired explicit permission to perform the service.

Unfortunately, even if insurance authorizes service, it will not guarantee payment to the provider. As a result of this, virtually all providers will ask you to sign an Advanced Beneficiary Notice (ABN) every time you go to see a physician or receive any type of treatment. An ABN basically says that if your insurance company does not pay, for any reason at all, that you agree to pay them instead. I have tried to see providers without agreeing to sign the ABN, and unfortunately, they usually turn me away.

This part of the system is susceptible to break-downs and there is plenty of blame to go around. Patients usually do not check the benefit plan for every single service they will receive. Similarly, insurance companies do not have the resources and talent available to allow them to assess the appropriateness of every single treatment prior to the time of service. So even if providers do get authorization to perform a service, the insurance company may still determine that the service was not appropriate after the fact. This is why healthcare providers reserve the right to collect unpaid balances from the patient. Payment is not guaranteed.

If worse comes to worst, you can ask the provider to switch your status to uninsured or self-pay and ask for the corresponding discount on charges. If you don't have benefits, then technically, you are uninsured.

Pre-existing medical conditions

This is a hot topic in the healthcare reform efforts of 2010 and may well be abolished by the time this book is published. It is also a complicated topic, so I am careful to explain it in a way that does not bias for or against any party. If you cannot get health insurance because of a pre-existing medical condition, I recommend that you contact the Foundation for Health Coverage Education (www. coverageforall.org) and they will direct you to a high-risk insurance pool in your state that will cover you. I am going to use an extreme example to explain pre-existing medical conditions.

If every person in the United States was enrolled in one giant health plan, everyone would pay a very similar premium. We would simply take the total cost of care for this year divided by the total number of people covered. Everyone would pay the same amount because it would be easy to calculate the total costs and the total number of people. Our sample size would include everyone. All of the actuaries would be unemployed.

However, we are not all enrolled in one plan. We are enrolled in thousands of different plans. Some of us are old and some of us are young. Some of us smoke and some of us do not. Some of us jump from one plan to another every year and some of us stay in the same plan for a decade. All of this makes it very difficult for each insurance company to predict what the total cost of care will be for their respective plans.

As a result of these factors, insurance companies may keep a list of "pre-existing medical conditions" that require that a new enrollee be put on a "waiting period" in which he or she has to pay premiums into the plan for several months before becoming eligible for treatment to be covered.

The Health Insurance Portability and Accountability Act (HIPAA) of 1997 factors into this as well. In accordance with HIPAA, a patient that finds new health insurance coverage within 63 days of the loss of their previous coverage may not be excluded for reason of pre-existing medical conditions. The purpose of this law is to dissuade people from going for long periods without coverage and to provide continuity of coverage for people who find new insurance quickly. HIPAA encourages people to stay covered all the time. Philosophically speaking, it is not fair to those who pay their premiums consistently if people only join when they get sick. If everyone was covered all the time, it would be much easier to predict the costs of care.

For example, let's assume that Irma is hired by your employer. Irma and her dependent husband have smoked for 25 years. Irma has emphysema and her husband has chronic obstructive pulmonary disease (COPD). Irma's entry into your employer's health plan will significantly elevate the cost of your premiums next year. The cost of her and her husband's care will far exceed the cost of many other employees combined. In effect, the rest of your company's employees will subsidize Irma's healthcare costs. So, to partially offset this inequity, the plan could require Irma to pay premiums into the plan for several months before she and her husband will have their care covered. The intent of the exclusion period is to offset the cost to your employer and everyone else in the plan. The intent is to make this change fair to everyone else. According to HIPAA, if Irma has joined within 63 days of the termination of her previous coverage then this exclusion period will not apply.

Here is another example that explains the other half of this. Let's assume that as Irma is joining your company's plan, Ted is leaving the plan. Ted developed heart disease last year and has been taking many new medications. Now that he is leaving the plan, the premiums of the group will decrease since the group is no longer paying for Ted's drugs. Should Ted have to wait six months before he can get coverage at his new job? According to HIPAA, if Ted finds new insurance coverage within 63 days of his last date of coverage, he cannot be excluded for pre-existing medical conditions. Again, the intent is for everyone to stay covered all the time. If everyone stays covered then most of these fluctuations should even out.

Not medically necessary

This type of denial places follow-up squarely on your provider, but I always encourage the patient to get involved. Insurance companies are essentially business people who follow general medical guidelines to manage the benefit process. The medical director of the insurance company is the only person who really makes medical judgments and he or she only reviews several dozen appeals each day.

The fact that you received this type of notice means that something about your treatment did not fit into the general policies programmed into the insurance company's claims system and the medical director has probably not seen it. These general policies are actually standardized across all insurance companies. They are called the Milliman's Medical Underwriting Guidelines and they are probably available on your insurance company's website. If they know what they're doing, your provider will find out which guideline is causing a problem and then issue an appeal that addresses the guideline as it relates to the uniqueness of your treatment.

Experimental treatment

If a treatment or device is approved by the Food & Drug Administration (FDA), generally the insurance companies will cover it as well. The insurance companies do not test the effectiveness of devices or treatments. They wait until there is sufficient research from medical colleges and universities and the FDA to make their coverage decision. After that point, it is up to your employer to decide whether it is to be included in your benefit plan. I'm not taking sides, but I would venture to say that new, cutting-edge treatments and drugs are most often not as effective for the patient as the traditional treatments. Don't misunderstand me, there are definitely legitimate advances, but they represent a minority, not the majority of experimental treatments.

THINGS TO KNOW IF YOU DON'T HAVE INSURANCE

This chapter covers public health insurance programs that are available as well as COBRA for those that have lost their jobs and an in-depth introduction to provider-based charity care. Charity care will be discussed in more detail in the following chapters.

If you don't have health insurance you still have good options and I'm confident that you'll be able to get access to quality medical care. Depending on your annual income and your number of dependents, you may have access to free medical care at many not-for-profit hospitals.

First, let's see if you are eligible for any public health insurance plans.

Medicare

Are you 65 years old or older? Do you have a permanent disability? Do you have end-stage renal disease?

Medicaid

Medicaid is a state program for the poor. What is great about Medicaid is that if you are eligible, you can get retro-active coverage, meaning *medical care you had 3 months ago can be covered if you apply today.*

State Children's Health Insurance Program

This is another great program that expands Medicaid for 4 million *children and pregnant women.*

In 2010, the Medicare, Medicaid, and State Children's Health Insurance Program (SCHIP) collectively cover about 30% of Americans. In the wake of the high unemployment of 2008 and 2009 and the 30 million baby boomers that will enroll in Medicare over the next seven years, I am confident that one out of every three Americans will be enrolled in one of these programs by 2017. It is because these programs have a large impact on so many people, that I have included content specifically to educate the reader because there is a one in three chance that you'll be enrolled in one of these programs in the next seven years.

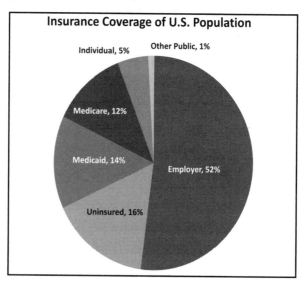

The U.S. healthcare "system" is a "hodge podge" of programs.

	Employer-Based Commercial Insurance	Privately Purchased Commercial Insurance	Public Insurance		
			Medicaid	SCHIP	Medicare
Birth - 6	Dependent of working parent covered by employer (must be in college if over 18)	Dependent of parent buying insurance directly from insurance company (must be in college if over 18)	Dependent of parent living in poverty for family size (<133% FPL)	Child dependent of parent living in poverty for family size (<200% FPL in 22 states) (>200% FPL in 28 states and D.C)	N/A Eligible if permanently disabled or have end-stage renal failure
Age 6-19			Dependent of parent living in poverty for family size (<100% FPL)		
Age 18-25			May be covered as dependent college student if state allows		
Age 25-65	Covered worker participating in employer-sponsored health plan	Buying insurance directly from insurance company	Eligible as adult relatives or legal guardians who take care of children under age 18 (or 19 if still in high school) (<60% FPL) or blind/disabled and receiving SSI	Covered if pregnant mother (<200% FPL in 22 states) (>200% FPL in 28 states and D.C.)	
Age 65-death	N/A	N/A	Maybe dually eligible as elderly in poverty. Medicaid will pay Medicare premiums.	N/A	Covered as elderly

Medicare

Medicare was created in 1965, when Congress and President Lyndon B. Johnson expanded FDR's social security program to include a social healthcare benefit for the elderly. Today, Medicare is the largest single health plan in the United States covering over 40 million people. By the year 2017, it is expected that over 70 million people will be enrolled in Medicare.

It is my opinion that Medicare is the best insurance plan in the United States. It offers a broad array of benefits at a very reasonable price to the enrollees. Commercial insurance companies copy everything Medicare does. All commercial insurance companies require medical providers to be Medicare certified before they can be included in their commercial health plans. Most commercial insurers only cover services covered by Medicare. When Medicare lowers or increases payment rates, commercial insurance will do the same.

The federal government only "underwrites" or pays for services under the Medicare program. The actual administration of the program is outsourced to commercial insurance companies that serve as "fiscal intermediaries" for Medicare. Fiscal intermediaries run the day-to-day logistics of benefit administration, while the federal government writes the checks. Fiscal intermediaries are middle men. Across the United States there are about a dozen insurance companies that serve as fiscal intermediaries or carriers that run day-to-day operations of the Medicare program. Every few years, the federal government accepts new "bids" and the fiscal intermediaries change.

Medicare has four major components lettered A-D.

1) Part A: Includes benefits for inpatient hospital care and post-acute care.

2) Part B: Includes benefits for outpatient services like physicians, imaging tests, minor surgery, etc.

3) Part C: Is called "Medicare Advantage" or "Medicare+Choice." This is the option to enroll in special Medicare plans that are

controlled more closely by commercial insurance companies. These are often cheaper than traditional Medicare. About 20% of Medicare enrollees have chosen Part C.

4) Part D: Includes prescription drug benefits. There are many different drug plans and formularies available.

To enroll in Medicare under the <u>elderly</u> benefit you have to meet the eligibility criteria.

- You must be a U.S. citizen or permanent resident

- You or your spouse must have worked 10 years at a job that deducted Medicare premiums from your pay

- You must be 65 years old or older

You can also enroll in Medicare if you have received social security benefits for a permanent disability for two years or if you have end-stage renal disease (kidney failure).

The retirement age to receive full social security benefits is now 67. However, Medicare enrollment is still age 65. You can begin the Medicare enrollment process three months before you turn 65. You benefits will start on the first day of the month of your 65th birthday. For example, if your birthday is April 15, then your Medicare benefits begin April 1. If your birthday happens fall on the first day of the month, then your Medicare benefits activate the first day of the month prior. In this case, if your birthday is March 1, your Medicare benefits will commence on February 1.

Medicare currently covers:

Medicare Part A covers inpatient and related medical care:

- Inpatient hospital care

- Skilled nursing facility care

- Home health care for post-acute medical needs of patients restricted to their homes

- Hospice care for the terminally ill

Medicare Part B covers outpatient medical care:

- Ambulance services

- Chiropractic care only for a manual subluxation of the spine

- Physician services

- Durable medical equipment

- Limited home health services

- Limited preventive care services

- Limited types of prescription drugs

- Outpatient mental health services

- Outpatient physical, speech, and occupational therapy services

- Radiology and lab tests

The Medicare Part D prescription drug benefit covers:

- Outpatient prescription drugs: Formulary (list of drugs covered) varies by the plan and insurance company you choose

Medicare does not cover:

- Alternative medicine like acupuncture and chiropractors

- Elective cosmetic surgery

- Dental

- Hearing aids

- Long-term care: defined as basic activities of daily living

- Some preventive care: most routine physicals, immunizations, and eye exams

Medicare managed care plans & HMOs:

These are Medicare plans run by commercial insurance companies that try to administer Medicare benefits cheaper than the government. These plans offer the same fundamental benefits as traditional Medicare, but may limit the providers you can see in an effort to keep costs down. The insurance company will likely restrict you to a network built around a group of very efficient, cost-effective medical providers to make this possible. You'll still have access to other providers in emergency situations.

You can save money by choosing a Medicare managed care plan over traditional Medicare, but be aware that you will have less choice when it comes to picking your medical providers. If you don't have loyalty to any specific physician, this could be a good option for you. I don't work for an insurance company and I am not a spokesperson for them, but I personally would have no problem limiting myself to fewer medical providers for a cheaper medical care. I'm not the type who will travel great distances for medical care.

Supplemental "Gap" Insurance:

You can purchase "gap" insurance from a private insurance company to supplement Medicare. Gap insurance will pay your Medicare deductibles, coinsurances, and copays. There are 12 different gap plans available for purchase, labeled alphabetically A to L.

Medicare premiums in 2010:

Part A: If you or your spouse has worked 10 years at a U.S. job that deducted Medicare from your pay, you do not pay a monthly Part A premium. The Medicare Part A premium is $254.00 per month for people who worked 7 ½ to 9 ¾ years in a U.S. job. The same premium is $461.00 per month for people who worked less than 7 ½ years in a U.S. job.

Part B: The Medicare Part B premium is $96.40 per month in 2010 for those already enrolled in Medicare whose incomes are less than $85,000 annually ($170,000 for couples). For new enrollees, the Medicare Part B monthly premium will be $110.50 in 2010, or even higher if your income is greater than $85,000 annually ($170,000 for couples).

Medicare deductibles and copays for 2010:

Part A: The Medicare Part A deductible is $1,100 in 2010. This covers the first 60 days of a hospital stay. I cannot emphasize what a fantastic deal this is, as hospital charges are usually $7,000-$10,000 per day. The patient must pay $275-$550 for each day spent at a hospital over 60 days up to 150 days. If the patient stays beyond 150 days, Medicare will pay all costs incurred beyond 150 days.

If the patient requires a stay at a skilled nursing facility, the first 20 days are paid by Medicare. The patient must pay $137.50 for each day from day 21 through day 100.

There is no deductible or copay for home health care after a hospital or skilled nursing facility stay.

Part B: The Medicare Part B deductible is $155 in 2010. There is a 20% coinsurance after meeting the deductible. This means that you'll have to pay 20% of the bill every time you go to see your physician.

Access to Medicare providers:

Some physicians have stopped seeing Medicare patients because they allege that payments are so low they lose money on every patient. This a small minority now, but I expect more physicians will do this in the future because Medicare payment rates will continue to go down and the percentage mix of all patient enrolled in Medicare is going to increase substantially. Though more solo practices may refuse Medicare, I'm confident the large physician groups will continue to see Medicare patients.

Medicaid

Medicaid is a federal program that "matches" money that states spend on health insurance for the very poor. About 47 million people were enrolled in Medicaid as of June of 2008. Over 70% of these people were enrolled in Medicaid "managed care" plans run by commercial insurance companies and health-maintenance organizations (HMOs).

Medicaid primarily helps provide health benefits for children in poor families and pregnant mothers. The State Children's Health Insurance Program (SCHIP) expands Medicaid's eligibility to reach more children. SCHIP is discussed in detail in the next section.

The poverty guidelines were originally written by an employee of the Social Security Administration in 1964. The SSA employee took the cost of the U.S. Department of Agriculture's economy food plan and multiplied that cost by three. This "three-times-food-cost" calculation was done in 1963 and every year since, the dollar amount has been increased for inflation by the Consumer Price Index of the current year. I suppose this is better than nothing, but I think most would agree that there must be a more equitable method of assessing poverty than the simple arithmetic method that was used almost 50 years ago.

Income and assets are the primary tests for Medicaid eligibility. It is possible that a person or family may be eligible for Medicaid health insurance, but not eligible for a traditional welfare program like Temporary Assistance for Needy Families (TANF). A person who may not qualify purely on an income basis, may still qualify for Medicaid if his or her medical expenses are "excessive."

The federal government established a minimum set of eligibility requirements for people who want to enroll in Medicaid. States must honor the minimum requirements. Fortunately, nearly all states have exercised their ability to expand the eligibility criteria beyond the minimum.

The federal government's minimum requirements are organized into several eligibility groups:

- Categorically needy

- Medically needy

- Special groups

The categorically needy are primarily defined as:

- Pregnant women and children under age six whose family income is at or below 133% of the Federal Poverty Level (FPL). The Medicaid program served 29 million children in 2006. Medicaid pays for a full set of services for children, including preventive care, screening and treatment of health conditions, physician and hospital visits, and vision and dental care. In most cases, these services are provided at little to no cost to the family.

- Children ages 6 to 19 with family income up to 100% of the FPL.

- Those receiving Supplemental Security Income (SSI) are generally automatically enrolled in Medicaid (primarily blind and disabled).

- Individuals and couples living in medical institutions with limited monthly income (primarily long-term care).

Medically needy:

This group has too much money or too much savings to be eligible as categorically needy. If a state chooses to provide a medically needy program, it must minimally include pregnant and recently pregnant women, newborns, children under age 18, and protected blind persons.

States may also elect to provide Medicaid to college students, as well as the aged, blind, and disabled. Over two-thirds of states include the aged, blind, and disabled as eligible under a medically needy program.

States Electing to Offer Medically Needy Programs					
Arkansas	Hawaii	Maine	Nebraska	Pennsylvania	Vermont
California	Illinois	Maryland	New Hampshire	Puerto Rico	Virginia
Connecticut	Iowa	Massachusetts	New Jersey	Rhode Island	Washington
D.C.	Kansas	Michigan	New York	Tennessee	West Virginia
Florida	Kentucky	Minnesota	North Carolina	Texas (limited)	Wisconsin
Georgia	Louisiana	Montana	North Dakota	Utah	

Special groups:

Medicare enrollees
Medicaid pays Medicare premiums, deductibles, copays, and coinsurance for those enrolled in Medicare that have income at or below 100% of the FPL and total personal savings less than 200% of the standard allowed under Supplemental Security Income (SSI). Medicare enrollees with income over 100% of FPL but less than 135% of FPL may also have limited Medicare cost-share responsibilities paid by Medicaid.

Working disabled on Medicare
Medicaid pays Medicare Part A premiums for the disabled individuals who would lose Medicare coverage because they work. Medicaid will pay Medicare Part A premiums if the disabled working person still has income below 200% of FPL and personal savings less than 200% of the standard SSI allowance.

Several states offer Medicaid for uninsured persons with specific diseases, regardless of income or assets. Forty-two states and the District of Columbia offer Medicaid to women who have breast or cervical cancer. Those states that provide Medicaid to persons infected with tuberculosis (TB) are listed in the following table.

States Electing to Offer Medicaid to Person with Tuberculosis			
California	Minnesota	Puerto Rico	Wisconsin
D.C	New York	Rhode Island	Wyoming
Louisiana	Oklahoma	Utah	

Medicaid managed care and HMOs

In the same way Medicare is administered by commercial insurance companies as a Medicare Advantage plan or through an HMO, many states offer Medicaid through commercial insurance companies and HMOs. States do this because commercial insurance companies are efficient at controlling excessive costs. They can run a Medicaid program more efficiently than state employees. Sometimes, the Medicaid HMOs and similar entities are so much cheaper that they can offer a broader range of service and benefits to Medicaid enrollees without materially increasing the overall cost of the program. This is a trade off. By enrolling in a Medicaid HMO or similar plan, you give up freedom of choice in exchange for a possible broader range of services.

Long-term care

Medicaid is the primary payer for most long-term care, including nursing homes and home care. At present, there is no long-term care benefit under the Medicare program. The Medicaid eligibility criteria usually require the patient/resident to "spend down" income and assets so that they will qualify for Medicaid. The process of liquefying and transferring assets is highly legal in nature, unique to each state, and beyond the scope of this book. If you are trying to enroll an elderly adult in Medicaid to pay for long-term care, I recommend that you contact your state's long-term care ombudsman or Medicaid ombudsman so that they can counsel you on the process.

State Children's Health Insurance Program

The State Children's Health Insurance Program (SCHIP) expands state Medicaid programs to cover children of parents who have too much money to be eligible for Medicaid, but likely not enough to buy commercial insurance. Check the state-specific information in the back of this book to find the expanded income levels for the SCHIP program in your state. Some states also allow families to "buy into" the SCHIP program at a reduced rate if they make too much income to be eligible on a regular basis. Benefits will be different in each state.

This chart illustrates how Medicaid and SCHIP work in tandem to cover various populations in my home state of Colorado. Different states use different percentages of FPL along the left axis. While the 100% is generally the bare minimum Medicaid eligibility level set by the federal government for children 6-19 years old, the two healthcare reform bills currently being considered in early 2010 would raise minimum coverage to 150% of FPL (HR 3962) or 133% of FPL (HR 3590). Both bills would make Medicaid accessible to a larger population of people.

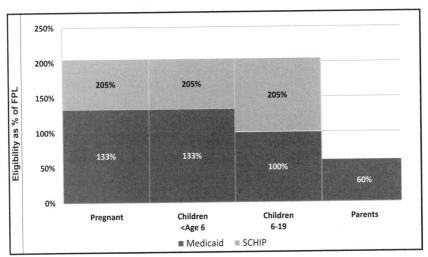

Colorado Medicaid and SCHIP

Did you lose your job?

The Consolidated Omnibus Budget Reconciliation Act of 1985 (COBRA) requires health plans to continue to offer insurance coverage to employees who have been terminated or "laid off."

The catch is that the employer is no longer obligated to pay the majority of the premiums. In fact, they will most likely pay nothing. It is all on the employee. Needless to say, the ability of the average person to pay 100% of a family's health insurance premiums is significantly impaired by the fact that he or she has just been let go. Failure to make the monthly premium payments by the ex-employee will result in the termination of coverage.

Fortunately, the American Recovery and Reinvestment Act of 2009, signed by President Obama on February 17, 2009, includes a 65% subsidy of health insurance premiums for ex-employees for up to 9 months if termination of employment occurred between September 1, 2008 and December 31, 2009. This means the federal government will pay 65% of your health insurance premiums. This is a great deal.

The Department of Defense Appropriations Act of 2010, signed by President Obama on December 21, 2009, extended the COBRA subsidy from nine months to fifteen months. It also extended the layoff eligibility date to those affected on or before February 28, 2010.

COBRA cannot require an insurer to continue to provide coverage if the employer drops group coverage or if the loss of employment is caused by the closing of the employer's business altogether.

There are several "qualifying events" that determine eligibility for COBRA coverage:

1) The loss of employer-based group health insurance coverage from voluntary resignation, reduction in hours below health insurance eligibility level, involuntary termination (except for

extreme adverse misconduct or behavior), layoff, strike, or prolonged illness and medical leave.

2) Divorce from a spouse who is the primary policyholder.

3) The death of the employee who is the primary policy holder.

4) A dependent child over 18 who is not enrolled in college or has exceeded the eligibility age while still in college.

If the qualifying event is divorce, then COBRA is available for up to 36 months after the event. COBRA is minimally available for 18 months after other qualifying events.

What type of provider did you see?

If you're uninsured, I advise you to become aware of the difference between not-for-profit providers and for-profit providers.

Most of the original "hospitals" in the U.S. were started by churches as charities for the sick and dying. In 1910, something called the Flexner Report was published, which had the effect of forcing physician specialists and university medical schools to "marry" themselves to hospitals where large numbers of sick people were located in one place. This was great for physicians because they no longer had to ride a horse all over town going from house to house.

Ironically, 100 years later, healthcare has become the fastest growing business segment of the U.S. economy and about 60% of community hospitals are still legally set up as church-sponsored charities or education-related charities. Both church-sponsored hospitals and university-based hospitals have a not-for-profit status.

If you are uninsured, this is great news for you. Though not-for-profit hospitals are bound by the broad-based definition of "health promotion" of the IRS, in the society we live in, they are still held to something called the charity care standard[1,2]. Not-for-profit hospitals have to provide "free" charity medical care or the IRS will slap huge penalties on them. What is also good for you is that it is becoming harder every year to be a physician and more and more of them are becoming employees of these not-for-profit hospitals. If you went to a Catholic, Presbyterian, Methodist, or Lutheran hospital, I'm confident that you are going to be just fine after you read Chapter 4. It is the same with university hospitals.

If you went to a for-profit hospital and are uninsured, this will be a little harder, but we'll get through it. I recommend you read Chapter 3 and Chapter 4 very thoroughly.

Generally speaking, if you're having trouble paying your bills and you can change your provider, I advise you to try to go to a not-for-profit hospital in the future. You can tell your physician this too. They can take you to any hospital you want if you tell them why.

In the past few years, not-for-profit hospitals have been under very close scrutiny when it comes to providing charity care to the uninsured. If you are genuinely experiencing hardship, and they refuse to work with you, the hospital faces major legal penalties. Over 400 class-action lawsuits have been filed by Richard Scruggs and ten other law firms against not-for-profit hospitals on behalf of uninsured patients, claiming that tax-exempt hospitals are not justifying their exemption because they bill uninsured and underinsured patients with full charges[3,4]. Setting fair discount levels is truly an ethical challenge for hospitals. Setting the discount levels too high will compromise the financial livelihood of the hospital while setting discount levels too low will prohibit some patient needs from being met.

---

1 Principles & Practice Board Examines the Relationship of Community Benefit to Hospital Tax-Exempt Status, Healthcare Financial Management Association, April 20, 2005.
2 Gundling, Richard L., A Taxing Question for Not-for-Profits, *Healthcare Financial Management*, August 2005.
3 Clarke, Richard L., Creating Community Connections, *Healthcare Financial Management*, October 2004.
4 Taylor, Mark, Scruggs gains in some states, *Modern Healthcare*, August 22, 2005, p 26.

There are several states on the forefront of ensuring medical care is available to the uninsured:

Minnesota

Minnesota is the central state in the community benefit debate. Minnesota Attorney General Mike Hatch threatened to file a suit against 110 Minnesota hospitals if they were non-compliant with a two-year contract he established with the Minnesota Hospital Association that set the level of required charity care at 5% of operating costs and established guidelines for collection practices. The collection practice guidelines force hospitals to give patients with net incomes less than $125,000 the "most favored" discount rate of each hospital's payers. This means that the uninsured in Minnesota get the same financial treatment as the patients with each hospital's best insurance contracts.

California

One out of five California citizens is uninsured (7 million) and another 3 million are underinsured. California hospitals provide $4 billion in uncompensated care annually. The guidelines established by the California Healthcare Association are uniquely vivid among guidelines established by other state hospital associations and the American Hospital Association[5]:

- "Fear of a hospital bill should never prevent any Californian from seeking emergency health care services."

- "Financial assistance provided by the hospital is not a substitute for personal responsibility."

- "Patients who are at or below 300% of the FPL are eligible to apply for financial assistance under each hospital charity care

5 California Hospital Billing and Collection Practices: Voluntary Principles and Guidelines for Assisting Low-Income Uninsured Patients, California Healthcare Association, February 6, 2004.

policy or discount payment policy."

- "... each hospital should limit expected payments from these patients ... to amounts that do not exceed the payment the hospital would receive from Medicare ..."

- "For patients who have an application pending for [financial assistance] a hospital should not knowingly send that patient's bill to a collection agency prior to 120 days from the time of the initial billing."

- "Any payment plans offered by a hospital ... in settling past due outstanding hospital bills shall be interest free."

- "The hospital or outside collection agency operating on behalf of the hospital shall not ... use wage garnishments or liens on primary residences as a means of collecting unpaid hospital bills."

Illinois

In February of 2004, the Illinois Department of Revenue withdrew the tax-exempt status of Provena Covenant Medical Center[6,7]. In September of 2006, the Illinois Department of Revenue re-affirmed the 2004 judgment. The director of the Illinois Department of Revenue based his decision on 2002 figures that reveal Covenant's revenues of $113 million and charitable activities of only $831,724 (only 0.7%). Covenant's argument that non-reimbursed costs of Medicare and Medicaid be counted as charity was denied.

The Director of Revenue quoted:

> *This small amount of charitable care is so seriously insufficient that it simply cannot withstand the constitutional scrutiny*

---

6 Maiuro, Lisa S., Endangered Species?, Not-for-Profit Hospitals Face Tax-exempt Challenge, *Healthcare Financial Management,* September 2004.
7 Illinois Not-for-Profit Hospital Loses Property Tax Exemption, HFMA News Brief, October 2, 2006.

required to justify a property tax exemption. And since 97.7% of Covenant's revenue "was generated from the exchange of services for payment," the hospital's property could not have been considered used exclusively for charitable purposes.

Provena appealed to Sangamon County Circuit Court which decided in favor of the health system in July of 2007. Then the Illinois Attorney General Lisa Madigan got really fired up and filed an appeal against Provena. The 4th District Appellate Court of Illinois decided against Provena in August of 2008. Provena appealed again to the Illinois Supreme Court, which should render a decision in early 2010.

GETTING ORGANIZED

Before we talk to billers, I want you to be very familiar with your financial situation and feel totally confident in what you are talking about. This chapter will show you how to organize and prepare for these important conversations. If you have already talked to billers and it didn't go well, that's okay. I'm going to teach you how to recover from any bad calls you've already had and how to try to mend your bridges if you've been sent to collections. Again, I want to get rid of your anxiety. If you just had a catastrophic medical episode, the last thing you need to be worried about is your bills. Trust me. It's going to be fine.

How to develop a system for tracking bills and payments and EOBs

If you've recently had a hospital stay or been admitted to a hospital through the emergency room, you are going to get several bills and they are not all going to be from the hospital. You are going to get bills from the emergency medicine physicians in the ER, the radiology group that read your x-rays and MRIs, the pathology group that analyzed your lab tests, the specialist physicians and surgeons who looked after you once you were admitted to the hospital, and the hospital facility itself. You may have follow-up office visits with a specialist, several types of ongoing treatments, physical therapy, or home care.

I know it's overwhelming and intimidating because this has never happened to you before. You were not planning for this, the bills keep coming in the mail, and you are afraid of what will happen when you run out of money.

I'm not telling you this to scare you and I'm not scared for you, because I have done this so often that I actually enjoy talking to billers and I hope to show you how easy it can be.

Before we ever talk to billers, we need to have a plan. On the opposite page you will see a template I made for you to help you get a handle on the range and scope of your liabilities. You can create a duplicate of this template or download it from the book's companion website at www.medicalbillsurvivalguide.com and fill it in to keep a record of all the correspondence between you and your providers and your insurance company.

How to use bills and EOBs to get control of your situation

For every service you have done, you will receive a bill from the provider and an Explanation of Benefits (EOB) from your insurance company. An EOB is a notice from the insurance company that tells you if the insurance company paid and what is due from the patient to the provider, if anything. If you do not have insurance, you will only receive the bill.

If you have insurance, it is very important that you keep track of all the bills and EOBs that you receive. Every service you have will have both a bill and an EOB. I recommend that you 1) staple matching bills and EOBs together, 2) file them in folders by provider, and 3) sort them by date of service. You can use the template on the opposite page as an index. It will help you keep track at a glance without having to dig through tons of papers.

Medical Bill Log - Template

Service Date	Bill Date	Bill Number	EOB Date	EOB #	Service Description	Insurance Paid?	Patient Amt Due?	Call Date	Biller Name	Comments

Diagram: Filing system for bills, statements, and EOBs

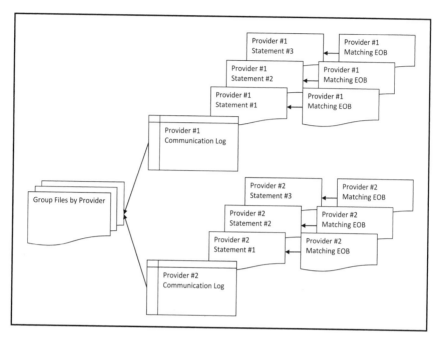

How to read a medical bill

Business management guru Peter Drucker once called U.S. hospitals the most complex organizations in human history. I regret that this is in no small part due to the complexity of the relationship between hospitals, patients, physicians, and insurance organizations.

On the opposite page is an example of a patient account statement for a wrist surgery performed on a Medicare enrollee. As you can see, the top line of the statement is over $14,000. An elderly patient receiving this statement might become distressed if he or she did not understand the rest of the statement. Just glancing at this statement one might also believe that the patient owed $388.20 to the facility. That is not the case. In fact, this patient owes nothing. There is a secondary insurance policy that has not yet paid, but will ultimately cover the balance of the amount owed.

Example: Patient statement

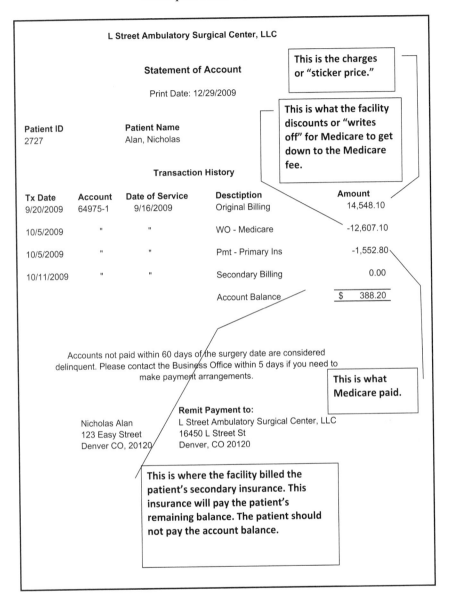

L Street Ambulatory Surgical Center, LLC

Statement of Account

Print Date: 12/29/2009

This is the charges or "sticker price."

This is what the facility discounts or "writes off" for Medicare to get down to the Medicare fee.

Patient ID	Patient Name
2727	Alan, Nicholas

Transaction History

Tx Date	Account	Date of Service	Desctiption	Amount
9/20/2009	64975-1	9/16/2009	Original Billing	14,548.10
10/5/2009	"	"	WO - Medicare	-12,607.10
10/5/2009	"	"	Pmt - Primary Ins	-1,552.80
10/11/2009	"	"	Secondary Billing	0.00
			Account Balance	$ 388.20

Accounts not paid within 60 days of the surgery date are considered delinquent. Please contact the Business Office within 5 days if you need to make payment arrangements.

This is what Medicare paid.

Nicholas Alan
123 Easy Street
Denver CO, 20120

Remit Payment to:
L Street Ambulatory Surgical Center, LLC
16450 L Street St
Denver, CO 20120

This is where the facility billed the patient's secondary insurance. This insurance will pay the patient's remaining balance. The patient should not pay the account balance.

What "charges" really mean in healthcare

When you get a bill from a healthcare provider there will be a line near the top called "charges" or "facility fee." It will be a big number, and this is what scares most people when they get a medical bill. Carol developed tunnel vision and only saw the numbers at the top of her bills. This is why she was in such a hurry to declare bankruptcy. This is a wrong way of thinking. I will use an analogy to explain why we do this.

Let's compare an MRI scan to getting a new transmission for your car. If ten different people take their car to the same body shop to get their transmission replaced, they are all going to pay the same thing. Let's say that bill is $900. Even though some will pay by check, some by cash, and some by credit card, they will all pay $900.

However, if ten different people go to the same hospital to get an MRI scan, their insurance companies are all going to pay different amounts and the patients are all going to pay different amounts. This is because:

- Insurance companies get "volume discounts" for the number of enrollees they cover. The more enrollees they have in their plan, the cheaper prices they can negotiate with healthcare providers. Providers will agree to lower rates, if being in the health plan means more patients will come see them. So a big insurance company like United Healthcare may negotiate a price for an MRI at, say, $1,000 while a smaller insurance company like Union Pacific Railroad Employee PPO might pay, say, $1,700 for the same MRI.

- Also, employers select different benefit plans within each insurance company based on what they can afford. Patients at Company A and Company B may both have United Health Insurance, but the patients at Company A could have a 20% coinsurance for an MRI while patients at Company B may have a 60% coinsurance for an MRI. This is purely a function of the plan your employer chooses.

Because there is no standard fixed price for medical service (like there is for transmissions) everybody pays something different. What's worse is that what everybody pays changes every year because employers, providers, and insurance companies re-negotiate every year. It is a real mess.

Providers don't want to keep 1,000 different price lists for all the different insurance companies, health plans, and employers. So what they do is keep one list, with very high "sticker prices" and just keep track of the 1,000 different types of discounts they have to apply to get down to the rates they agreed to in their contracts. These sticker prices are called "charges" or "facility fee" and that is all they are—sticker prices.

What "insurance discount" or "contractual allowance" means

The volume discounts I mentioned show up on the bills as "insurance discount" or "contractual allowance." This is a reduction that is applied to reach the rate agreed in the provider-insurance contracts. If you do not have insurance, providers will not stick you with a full sticker price for being uninsured. They will apply an "uninsured discount" that is often significant. At the surgery center that I ran, one of our largest discounts was our "uninsured discount" at 70% of charges. That means our uninsured patients only paid 30% of sticker price. If they applied for financial assistance, some would get even more discounts.

Itemized vs. unitemized

If you stay overnight in a hospital, they are going to mail you a free book in the mail. That book is your itemized bill. It will detail every charge and discount for every single billable procedure, supply, bandage, suture, gown, meal, and room fee you can imagine. Fortunately, your insurance company will bundle all of these things together in one payment. Some providers will send you an unitemized bill that has four lines: charges, insurance discount, insurance payment, and balance due. If the balance due is questionable, ask for an itemized bill.

Deductibles, copays, and coinsurance

We discussed these in Chapter 1, but to recap, the insurance company will always apply your deductible first before they start paying bills. Your copays are fixed amounts you pay for different types of visits and coinsurance is a percentage you pay for different types of visits. If you cannot afford to pay these, you may have options depending on your annual income, number of dependents, and total annual medical costs. We will jump into this in the next chapter.

Days delinquent, last payment, new charges

There are other parts of the bill you should note:

Days delinquent or outstanding

If your bill is less than 60 days outstanding, you are in good shape. If it is 60-90 days outstanding, you may be flirting trouble. At 90-120 days, your account is eligible for collections. At over 120 days, I would say a call from a collection agency is inevitable.

Last payment

It is good to note that the provider is receiving and posting your payments to your account. Billing offices that are understaffed may be a week or more behind in posting payments — not to mention the two or three days for U.S. Postal Service. If your monthly statement does not include a recent payment you made, call the provider and tell them when you mailed it and the check number and amount. They will put a note on your account and they will appreciate the call.

New charges

Most providers will send you a new statement every 30 days, or immediately after there is new activity. If you are seeing the same provider over and over, make new entries in your table to keep track of different dates of service. It can become very confusing to keep track of all the copays when you see the same specialist every two weeks for several months. You can accumulate numerous bills.

How to read an EOB

As I mentioned before, the Explanation of Benefits (EOB) is a notice from the insurance company that tells you if the insurance company paid and what is due from the patient to the provider, if anything. Every insurance company uses EOBs. They send them to the patient and to the provider. Be sure to reference the EOB when you talk to a biller.

This is a real EOB from my insurance company for an office visit I had with a physician specialist. You can see that the date of service was September 22, 2009. The charge or "sticker price" was $170. The insurance company allowed $145.60. This means the "insurance discount" was $24.40. I had a $25 copay for specialist office visits, so the insurance company paid the difference between the allowed amount ($145.60) and my copay of $25. $170 sticker price - $24.40 insurance discount = $145.60 allowed amount. $145.60 allowed - $25 copay = $120.60 insurance company payment.

NICHOLAS NEWSAD
4020 ROSEDALE PLAIN CITY RD
PLAIN CITY OH   43064

EXPLANATION OF BENEFITS

SERVICE DETAIL

PATIENT/RELAT CLAIM NUMBER	PROVIDER/ SERVICE	DATE OF SERVICE	AMOUNT CHARGED	NOT COVERED	AMOUNT ALLOWED	COPAY/ DEDUCTIBLE	PLAN COVERS	BENEFIT AVAILABLE	REMARK CODE
NICHOLAS 9663835101	EE D BARCZ OFFICE VISITS	09/22/09 TOTAL	170.00 170.00		145.60 145.60	25.00 25.00	100%	120.60* 120.60	D1
						PLAN PAYS		120.60	
						** PATIENT PAYS		25.00	

(*) INDICATES PAYMENT ASSIGNED TO PROVIDER

** DEFINITION: "PATIENT PAYS" IS THE AMOUNT, IF ANY, OWED YOUR PROVIDER. THIS MAY INCLUDE AMOUNTS ALREADY PAID TO YOUR PROVIDER AT TIME OF SERVICE.

REMARK CODE(S) LISTED BELOW ARE REFERENCED IN THE "SERVICE DETAIL" SECTION UNDER THE HEADING "REMARK CODE"
(D1) THANK YOU FOR USING A NETWORK PHYSICIAN OR OTHER HEALTH CARE PROFESSIONAL. WE HAVE APPLIED THE CONTRACTED FEE. THE PATIENT IS NOT RESPONSIBLE FOR THE DIFFERENCE BETWEEN THE AMOUNT CHARGED BY THE PHYSICIAN OR HEALTH CARE PROFESSIONAL AND THE AMOUNT ALLOWED BY THE CONTRACT, EXCEPT IN SITUATIONS WHERE THERE IS AN ANNUAL BENEFIT MAXIMUM FOR THIS SERVICE. THE PATIENT IS ALSO RESPONSIBLE FOR ANY COPAY, DEDUCTIBLE AND COINSURANCE AMOUNTS.

BENEFIT PLAN PAYMENT SUMMARY INFORMATION

D BARCZ	$120.60

SATISFIED 2009 TO-DATE	IN NETWORK DEDUCTIBLE	IN NETWORK OUT OF POCKET	OUT OF NETWORK DEDUCTIBLE	OUT OF NETWORK OUT OF POCKET
FAMILY NICHOLAS EE	$0.00 $0.00	$0.00 $0.00	$0.00 $0.00	$0.00 $0.00
PLAN YEAR 2009	FAMILY: $2000.00 INDIV: $1000.00	FAMILY: $6000.00 INDIV: $3000.00	FAMILY: $6000.00 INDIV: $3000.00	FAMILY: $12000.00 INDIV: $6000.00

A REVIEW OF THIS BENEFIT DETERMINATION MAY BE REQUESTED BY SUBMITTING YOUR APPEAL TO US IN WRITING AT THE FOLLOWING ADDRESS: UNITEDHEALTHCARE APPEALS, P.O. BOX 30432, SALT LAKE CITY, UT 84130-0432. THE REQUEST FOR YOUR REVIEW MUST BE MADE WITHIN 180 DAYS FROM THE DATE YOU RECEIVE THIS STATEMENT. IF YOU REQUEST A REVIEW OF YOUR CLAIM DENIAL, WE WILL COMPLETE OUR REVIEW NOT LATER THAN 30 DAYS AFTER WE RECEIVE YOUR REQUEST FOR REVIEW.

YOU MAY HAVE THE RIGHT TO FILE A CIVIL ACTION UNDER ERISA IF ALL REQUIRED REVIEWS OF YOUR CLAIM HAVE BEEN COMPLETED.

* * * * * * *

YOU CAN MEET MANY OF YOUR NEEDS ONLINE AT WWW.MYUHC.COM. AT ALMOST ANYTIME DAY OR NIGHT, YOU CAN REVIEW CLAIMS, CHECK ELIGIBILITY, LOCATE A NETWORK PHYSICIAN, REQUEST AN ID CARD, REFILL PRESCRIPTIONS IF ELIGIBLE, AND MORE! FOR IMMEDIATE, SECURE SELF-SERVICE, VISIT WWW.MYUHC.COM.

HOW TO REGISTER?
YOU CAN REGISTER AND BEGIN USING MYUHC IN THE SAME SESSION. ACCESS WWW.MYUHC.COM TO REGISTER. THE INFORMATION REQUIRED IS ON YOUR INSURANCE ID CARD (FIRST NAME, LAST NAME, MEMBER ID, GROUP NUMBER AND DATE OF BIRTH).
* * * * * * *

MAINTAINING THE PRIVACY AND SECURITY OF INDIVIDUALS' PERSONAL INFORMATION IS VERY IMPORTANT TO US AT UNITEDHEALTHCARE. TO PROTECT YOUR PRIVACY, WE HAVE IMPLEMENTED STRICT CONFIDENTIALITY PRACTICES. THESE PRACTICES INCLUDE THE ABILITY TO USE A UNIQUE INDIVIDUAL IDENTIFIER. YOU MAY SEE THE UNIQUE INDIVIDUAL IDENTIFIER ON UNITEDHEALTHCARE CORRESPONDENCE, INCLUDING MEDICAL ID CARDS (IF APPLICABLE), LETTERS, EXPLANATION OF BENEFITS (EOBS) AND PROVIDER REMITTANCE ADVICES (PRAS). IF YOU HAVE ANY QUESTIONS ABOUT THE UNIQUE INDIVIDUAL IDENTIFIER OR ITS USE, PLEASE CONTACT YOUR CUSTOMER CARE PROFESSIONAL AT THE NUMBER SHOWN AT THE TOP OF THIS STATEMENT.

THIS IS NOT A BILL

Putting it together

The provider bill and insurance EOB are two sides of the same story. There are two important things to check with each pair of bills and EOBs:

> Do your bills match up with your EOB? Do charges, discounts, and patient responsibilities match? They should. If not, you can ask the provider to conference call you and your insurance company together so they can hash it out. Definitely do this if the patient responsibility on the medical bill and the EOB do not match. The provider cannot bill you for more than the patient responsibility on the EOB. Once the conference call starts and you have voiced your concern, just listen while they work it out.

> Was the provider paid or not? Why? Some providers get into the habit of forwarding a bill to the patient if they are having trouble with an insurance company. If you are getting calls from a biller, it may be because they need to check your birth date or policy number. Don't be afraid to take a biller's phone call. If the insurance company is not paying there is a reason, and it is best to find out what the reason is a soon as possible.

HOW TO TALK TO BILLERS PRODUCTIVELY

It is important that you're prepared to talk to a biller when he or she calls. If someone calls and you are not prepared, tell them the truth and say you need time to get organized and understand your bills first. The billers definitely take time to know your account before they call (although some now use automated dialing). Before you talk, you need to fill out the template in the previous chapter and know the total amount owed from all providers as well as what is expected in the foreseeable future.

The difference between billers and collection agencies

A "biller" is an employee of the provider that you saw for treatment. This person works for the physician or hospital to process their bills and post payments as they come in. A "collector" is from a collection agency and is not an employee of the provider. Collectors get involved after your account is 90-120 delinquent. Billers will mark your account as "bad debt" to get it off their books and then forward your account to collections. Here is the key: billers only send your account to collections if they believe that you are *able, but not willing* to pay your bills. Collectors can be aggressive and intimidating. They can adversely affect your credit score or place liens on your home or property if you do not pay your bills.

The American Hospital Association, the California Healthcare Association, and the Hospital and Health System Association of Pennsylvania have all published that hospitals should have written policies that establish when and under whose authority patient debt is advanced for collection. The American Hospital Association says that hospitals are responsible for establishing the standard for debt collection with third party collectors and that the hospitals are ultimately responsible for the actions of the collector. All hospitals should have some level of supervision over their collection agency. The collection agency should not have the authority to sue on their own accord without approval from the hospital.

Why you want to stay out of collections

You do not want to be sent to collections. When you're dealing with a biller you have many options. They can setup payment plans and you can apply for financial aid. You can get deferments and in some cases, you can develop rapport and possibly get bills for some services waived. You don't have any of these options when you are sent to collections. If you were already sent to collections before you picked up this book, we have to get the biller to reverse their bad debt write-off. This is the most difficult thing that I'll teach you to do and I am saving it for last. First, I want you to understand how billers think and how to talk to billers.

Who billers are

I want you to get a feel for a day in the life of a biller. Billers may work a slightly later schedule than the normal 8-5 day because they are better able to reach people at home in the evenings. They do not like to call people at work if they can avoid it. If they call you in the morning, that means they want to leave you a message and that they don't necessarily need to speak to you directly.

Each biller will monitor 500 to 800 accounts per month. If you do the arithmetic, that means they have to make 20-35 calls per day to reach everyone once a month. That means they only want to spend five to ten minutes on each call per day. An account holder that keeps a biller on the phone for a half hour telling a sob story can become very irritating to a biller because the biller now has to stay later to finish his or her calls. If you call them, they will first spend a few seconds reviewing your account, checking to see what kind of insurance you have, how old your account is, what you had done, and most importantly, what the notes on your account say. I will discuss this in more detail, but good notes on your account can greatly improve your situation.

Most calls *from billers* are for one of three different things:

Something went wrong with your insurance company. If you're getting calls from a biller, it may be because they need to check your birth date or policy number. If you purposely ignore billers they may have no choice but to eventually switch the whole amount from your insurance company to your name and possibly send your account to collections. It is a terrible tragedy when this happens, because a two to three minute clarification on insurance information can clear the whole thing up instantly.

They are calling to let you know your insurance company has paid and your patient responsibility is now due. This is not a collection call and they do not necessarily need the money today. It is just a reminder call.

Your account is over 60 days delinquent and they want to know what is wrong. They just want to know *why* they have not heard from you or seen any payments. If there is a legitimate reason for the delay, they will give you more time, set-up a payment plan, or waive parts of your balance. If you're experiencing hardship, the key is to clearly communicate your difficulty as I will demonstrate in the next few pages. If they don't hear from you, then they have no information and have no option but to send the account to collections. Some patients that qualify for assistance are not getting it only because they fail to produce a pay stub, tax return, bank information, or photo identification.[8]

---

8 Acts of Charity: Charity Care Strategies for Hospitals in a Changing Landscape, PriceWater-HouseCoopers Healthcare Research Institute, 2005.

Five Things Not to Say to a Biller

Here are five things that will damage your relationship with a biller. Some will merely annoy the biller and some will damage your credibility as an account holder who is willing to cooperate.

1) Don't say that the price is unreasonably high. This quickly becomes a philosophical argument. We do not have the ammunition to win this battle. If you have comparable charges from three to four competing medical facilities in the same market for the same service and the price you are disputing is clearly more than 10% higher than competitors, then you might have a basis for this argument. Huge insurance companies have teams of negotiators that argue that prices are too high all day long. These negotiators bring hoards of data and experience to the table and sometimes they still get stonewalled. This is what it takes to justify that prices are too high.

2) Don't dispute minor details like the exact number of statements or phone calls that you have received from the billing department. This type of hair splitting is not productive, and will earn you a reputation as being belligerent and argumentative. You don't want to be perceived as argumentative by the person who has authority to change your circumstances. You want to be perceived as cooperative.

3) Don't swear, be sarcastic, or insult the biller. You don't have to be happy or chipper either. Use an objective tone of voice. A sarcastic tone of voice or profanity will result in negative comments on the account notes. This type of behavior is not tolerated. Billers do not want to deal with account holders that are vulgar and abusive to them. If you swear on the phone with a biller, you'll have about a 60% chance that they will switch your account to collections immediately after hanging up.

4) Don't say that you *should not have to* pay your bill because of a minor service quality issue. If you do not have the ability to pay, *tell them the truth*. You don't have to make up excuses because

you cannot afford to pay. I have found that many patients that cannot afford to pay will sidestep the issue or make up excuses. Common excuses include:

- The facility was dirty
- The staff rushed me out
- I hardly spoke to or saw a physician

Significant medical quality issues may warrant a price reduction but major quality issues are "never events" like a wrong-site surgery or a hospital-acquired infection. These are things that should never happen, like operating on the wrong leg.

5) Don't share your personal problems. The biller doesn't need to know if you or an immediate family member has a drinking, drug, or depression problem. They don't need to know that you have to choose daily between buying food and your hospital bill or that you are going to declare bankruptcy. If you are truly unable to pay your bill, and you have told them, you are going to get financial aid. Billers can quantify the figures on tax returns and pay stubs. This is what they want. Unfortunately, they tend to get tons of information that they cannot quantify in the form of sob stories and immeasurable embellishments.

If you're in the middle of a catastrophic episode of cancer and you have a physician's note that says you cannot go to work, that is relevant to your inability to pay your bills because it affects your income and your ability to go back to work. This is worth mentioning.

There is no discount for getting the biller to feel sorry for you. It is not going to help you to embellish your story or try to negotiate with sympathy. Billers are looking for very specific things, and personal drama is not one of them. This may seem a little harsh, but the rules of billing and collections are pretty cut and dry. Either you qualify for financial aid or you do not. There is no prize for the saddest story or the best philosophical argument.

Inability to pay vs. unwillingness to pay

Billers are always trying to discern the difference between those who are *unable* to pay and those who are *unwilling* to pay. The more certain they are that someone is unable to pay, the more likely they will set up payment plans, give discounts, and waive balances[9]. The more certain they are that someone is unwilling to pay, the more likely the account will go to collections. As I said earlier, not-for-profit hospitals have to provide charity medical care in the form of free care and write-offs or the IRS will slap huge penalties on them. And because so many physicians are becoming employees of these not-for-profit hospitals, the same rules are starting to apply for physician bills as well. They can and will do this, but they have to have some evidence of inability.

Five things billers look for

1) Does this patient take and return our phone calls? You want the biller to view you as responsive and cooperative. Conversely, you absolutely don't want to be viewed as non-responsive and uncooperative. If you have a message from a biller, return the call, even if it is just to tell them that you need time to understand your bills. If you see your biller's number on caller ID, answer the phone. Do not ignore their calls hoping they will just go away. It is just as bad as ignoring the symptoms of a disease. It will not go away; it will just get worse.

2) What do the notes on the account say? The notes on your account can save or destroy your chances to get a break. The best advocates you will have are the positive comments from another biller. Things like "called back promptly," "good demeanor," and "called to verified payment received" are all positive things to have on your account notes.

3) Has this patient been uncivil or caused problems in the past? Getting angry on the phone will get you sent to collections. Insulting the biller or being sarcastic are completely counter-productive and

---

9 Hospitals Share Insights to Improve Financial Policies for Uninsured and Underinsured Patients: A Report from HFMA's *Patient Friendly Billing* Project, February 2005.

will hurt you. As a medical facility manager, I would never give a break to someone who was uncivil, mean, or vulgar to one of our billers. I remember a story that perfectly exemplifies this effect:

A patient I will call George had recently had a catastrophic medical episode and had spent several nights in the hospital. After he was sent home for several weeks, he came to our facility to have a follow-up outpatient surgery. George's wife received their first bill and promptly sent a payment for half of their coinsurance amount. Within a few days, she received two more statements from us and neither had noted her payment. George's wife was furious. She called one of our billers, a little old white haired woman named Patty, and berated and insulted Patty until she was in tears for "being incompetent and working at such an (expletive) place." Patty was devastated, both from being overworked and underappreciated.

Here is what happened. The medical facility I worked for was having a very challenging year and had just lost several employees to an aggressive competitor that was hiring them away. The company was understaffed and many of the personnel were working overtime to try to post payments to patients' accounts that were several weeks old. What had happened to George was that after his service, our system generated a bill and mailed it to him. Several days later his insurance company paid. This triggered an "activity" and generated another statement. A few days later marked 30 days since his service, causing another statement to be automatically generated and mailed. All the while, our company was behind in posting her payment to the account.

I was happy to learn that George's wife called back shortly, also in tears, and apologized profusely to Patty. George and she had been through a horrible ordeal and she was emotionally exhausted from trying to sort through the hospital bills. Our little error was simply the straw that broke the camel's back.

In calling back and explaining her frustration, George's

wife completely absolved herself. We were not going to send her to collections anyway, but I think this example perfectly illustrates the situation in which we often find ourselves.

4) Has this patient made an effort to pay his or her bills? How many days delinquent is the account? The key word here is "effort." Has the patient made any effort at all? A patient who has sent in $15 each month for four months on a $300 account is going to get better consideration than someone who has paid zero per month for four months.

I was more aggressive than most billers in that I wanted all accounts paid within six months. I would usually allow "micro-payments" the first few months if the patient would agree to a balloon payment at month six. Most billers will allow payment plans greater than six months. As a patient advocate, the longest payment terms I have ever gotten for someone was two years.

5) Has this patient followed an agreed upon payment plan? If you get the biller to agree to let you make payments, it is crucial that you not miss a payment. There is an "implied contract" when you enter a payment plan that the provider has waived its ability to collect the full amount due immediately as long as you make your payments on time. Once you miss a payment, this "implied contract" is breached and they can call the full amount due immediately. If you think you are going to miss a payment, I strongly recommend that you call the provider *before* the due date and let them know. This might be your only chance of preserving your payment plan.

How to talk to a biller

Now that we understand our bills and EOBs and we know how billers think, we are almost ready to talk to them. Let's suppose there's a biller on the phone. After the biller has introduced himself or herself and had a chance to ask any minor questions about your insurance or identity, I usually like to open with something like this:

I was happy with the service we received at your facility. They did a good job. I want to let you know that we fully intend to pay this bill, you guys did a great job taking care of me (or my father, etc.) and I really appreciate it. But if you have a minute or two there are a few questions I want to ask you to make sure I understand all of this.

Naturally, the biller will agree to answer your question. I like to phrase it this way because it conveys that you are cognizant and respectful of their time. At this point, I recommend giving one sentence of context, not your whole life story. Remember that billers have to make 20-35 calls per day and they covet their time. They will be appreciative if you value their time.

To give you just a little context, I (or my father, uncle, etc.) just had a catastrophic episode of cancer and we are working with ten different providers to set-up payment plans and financial aid so everyone can get paid.

This lets them know your circumstances and that you are making efforts to meet *all of your obligations*, including theirs. At this point, you can open with logistical questions like why is there a discrepancy between their bill and your EOB, or try to figure out why your insurance did not pay. Ask for a conference call with your insurance company. That will allow you to get discrepancies resolved immediately rather than waiting for the biller to take care of it. After you have dealt with these issues, you are ready to talk about payment plans and financial aid.

Five things that every biller will consider

These following five strategies are really the crux of this book. Depending on your situation, you may be able to use a combination of these or all simultaneously. If you are genuinely experiencing hardship, these five strategies will help you demonstrate it in a rational manner to the provider. I do not condone lying or providing false information to try to get a break.

1) Payment plans

   Can I make payments of $xx per month?

   Payment plans are the simplest and easiest form of financial aid to get. Hospitals and healthcare providers will not charge you interest or penalties. It is highly frowned upon. You can usually get payment plans with or without insurance coverage. You can probably get a payment plan upon request if you ask for four months or less. If it is four months or more that you request, they will probably want to see you demonstrate hardship in the form of total medical costs or some measure of inability to pay for lack of personal income.

You can also lock in a payment plan early to avoid being sent to a collection agency. If you do get a payment plan setup, don't miss a payment without calling in advance or risk breaking the implied contract. When you agree to a payment plan, there is an implied contract wherein the provider is waiving its right to collect payment immediately as long as you agree to make payments according to the agreed plan you discuss.

This is just semantics, but I don't recommend generally asking, *"Can I make monthly payments?"* or asking the biller *"What is the smallest payment I can make?"* While the biller can be your friend, he or she is still incented to get the highest payments possible and to collect as much of your account balance as possible. I suggest that you propose the first dollar amount to them and pick a number that is comfortably low so that things could go wrong in your life and you can still make your monthly payment.

If you owe *more* than $500 on any one account and you are experiencing significant financial hardship, I recommend opening up with a monthly payment equal to 1/24th of what you owe. Do this arithmetic yourself and give them the dollar figure, do not say, *"Can I make 24 payments?"* Instead, say, *"Can I please make payments of $25 per month?"* They may come back with a higher dollar number or shorter term, but that is okay, because you set the initial bar very low. If they take it, be very happy.

Some organization will ask for your tax return just to qualify you for a simple payment plan. I think this is overkill. If they do this, ask them to "freeze" your account while you mail in your financial aid application.

There is not a bank in the U.S. that would loan you money for 24 months at an interest rate less than 7%-8%. If you had an introductory interest-free offer on a credit card, it would only last six to twelve months.

2) Poverty

The Federal Poverty Level (FPL) is the most common proxy for financial aid consideration. Nearly all hospitals employ some variation of a sliding scale discount in which the discount increases as the patient's income decreases relative to the FPL. Again, billers can be your friends, but because they're incented to collect as much as they can, they will probably not advertise their charity care policies upfront. You will have to initiate this conversation yourself.

The 2010 Poverty Guidelines

Persons in family	48 States	Alaska	Hawaii
1	$10,830	$13,530	$12,460
2	14,570	18,210	16,760
3	18,310	22,890	21,060
4	22,050	27,570	25,360
5	25,790	32,250	29,660
6	29,530	36,930	33,960
7	33,270	41,610	38,260
8	37,010	46,290	42,560
Add $3,740 for each additional person.		Add $4,680 for each person.	Add $4,300 for each person.

Source: http://www.cms.hhs.gov/MedicaidEligibility/Downloads/POV10Combo.pdf

This is how they work:

Someone earning less than 200% of the FPL might be eligible for a 100% discount while someone at less than 300% of the FPL might only be eligible for a 50% discount. If you make less than 400% of FPL, you might get 25% off charges. The great news is that, FPL is not a fixed number. The more dependents you have, the higher the FPL level is. If you talk to the right person, they will give you these discounts on this basis whether you have insurance or not.

You will have to verify your income and dependents for them. They will need your most recent tax return and your last two pay stubs.

The table on the previous page outlines 100% of the FPL for families of various sizes. If you make less than 400% of FPL for your family size, you definitely should mention it to your biller. Also, I strongly recommend that you communicate this in terms of your adjusted gross income (AGI) after your payroll deductions. Do not use your gross income. This is not your high school reunion. You are not trying to impress the biller with how much you make. You can see that AGI is found on line 4 of the 1040EZ form on the opposite page.

I once had a pastor with six children who wanted to pay for a surgery for one of his sons. He called me ahead of time and arranged a time to bring in his last tax return and two most recent pay stubs. His adjusted gross income was less than $20,000 a year. For his family size, he made less than 70% of FPL and he received a 90% discount. He was obviously well aware of his options and had done his homework. I was impressed.

Department of the Treasury—Internal Revenue Service

Form 1040EZ

Income Tax Return for Single and Joint Filers With No Dependents (99) 2009

OMB No. 1545-0074

Label
(See page 9.)

Use the IRS label.

Otherwise, please print or type.

Presidential Election Campaign (see page 9)

L A B E L	Your first name and initial	Last name		Your social security number
	If a joint return, spouse's first name and initial	Last name		Spouse's social security number
H E R E	Home address (number and street). If you have a P.O. box, see page 9.		Apt. no.	▲ You **must** enter your SSN(s) above. ◀
	City, town or post office, state, and ZIP code. If you have a foreign address, see page 9.			

▶ Checking a box below will not change your tax or refund.

Check here if you, or your spouse if a joint return, want $3 to go to this fund . . ▶ ☐ **You** ☐ **Spouse**

Income

Attach Form(s) W-2 here.

Enclose, but do not attach, any payment.

1 Wages, salaries, and tips. This should be shown in box 1 of your Form(s) W-2. Attach your Form(s) W-2. `1`

2 Taxable interest. If the total is over $1,500, you cannot use Form 1040EZ. `2`

3 Unemployment compensation in excess of $2,400 per recipient and Alaska Permanent Fund dividends (see page 11). `3`

4 Add lines 1, 2, and 3. This is your **adjusted gross income.** `4`

5 If someone can claim you (or your spouse if a joint return) as a dependent, check the applicable box(es) below and enter the amount from the worksheet on back.

☐ **You** ☐ **Spouse**

If no one can claim you (or your spouse if a joint return), enter $9,350 if **single;**

You may benefit from filing Form 1040A or 1040. See *Before You Begin* on page 4.

Sliding Income Scale

Persons in family	100% FPL	200% FPL	300% FPL	400% FPL
1	$10,830	$21,660	$32,490	$43,320
2	$14,570	$29,140	$43,710	$58,280
3	$18,310	$36,620	$54,930	$73,240
4	$22,050	$44,100	$66,150	$88,200
5	$25,790	$51,580	$77,370	$103,160
6	$29,530	$59,060	$88,590	$118,120
7	$33,270	$66,540	$99,810	$133,080
8	$37,010	$74,020	$111,030	$148,040

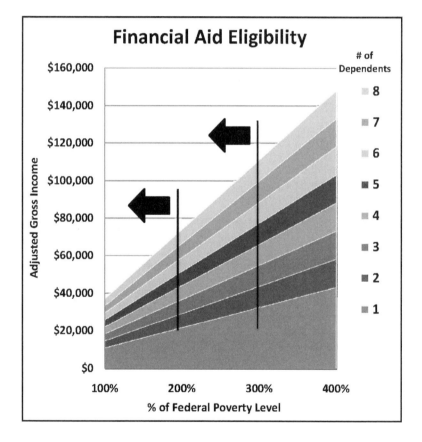

Federal Poverty Level	Catholic Healthcare West	Adventist Health	Providence Health System	Sutter Health	St Joseph Health System
Up to 200%	Free care	Free care	Free care	Free care	Free care
201-300%	Sliding scale not to exceed Medicare	75% discount on charges	Sliding scale not to exceed Medicare	Discounted to Medicare +20%, not to exceed 30% of household income	Sliding scale not to exceed Medicare
301%-350%	Average rate paid by largest insurance company	50% discount on charges	Sliding scale, not to exceed insurance company rates and based on overall need		Average insurance company rate
351%-400%		25% discount on charges			
401%-500%		N/A or case-by-case		N/A or case-by-case	
>501%	Case-by-case discounts based on circumstances				Case-by-case discounts based on circumstances

Source:http://www.nonprofithealthcare.org/resources/CA%20Hospital%20Systems-Charity%20Care%20Matrix.pdf

My family is another good example. I was one of four children. So, my dad had six dependents including my mom and the four kids. I am confident that for most of our childhood, Dad's adjusted gross income (AGI) would have fallen between 200% and 300% of poverty level. Dad made a good living, but Mom did not work and he had a modestly large family. If he had known the rules, he probably would have been eligible for a 25%-50% discount whenever we needed medical care.

Many hospitals and health providers employ a standard 10%-100% discount scale that fluctuates relative to the patient's income up to 400% of the FPL. Above is a table outlining the sliding scale discounts at the largest health systems in the state of California.

3) Catastrophic medical episode

The previous strategy uses FPL to demonstrate a patient's inability to pay. This strategy demonstrates inability to pay, by showing that a person's medical bills will consume a significant portion of their annual income. This is where the medical expense table in the previous chapter comes in handy. You need to have a running total of everything you owe on your medical bills and what new expenses you expect to incur in the next 12 months. Again, if you talk to the right person, he or she will consider discounts whether you have insurance or not. For example:

> *Let's say you make $100,000 per year and your annual adjusted gross income is $73,000. You have health insurance; however, you have a high deductible health plan with a $5,000 deductible and 40% coinsurance. You have a heart attack and are admitted to the hospital through the ER. You have two stents put in your heart immediately and return several months later to have a quadruple by-pass surgery. The two hospital admissions, cardiac catheterization, major surgery, and all the copays on the drugs you are now taking have racked up a total patient responsibility this year of $19,000. So, when you talk to the biller, you say, "My medical bills are going to be 26% of my adjusted gross income this year and this will cause significant hardship. I have copies of all my bills and my most recent tax return, am I eligible for financial aid?"*

Some hospitals will work out special plans to prevent medical expenses from ever exceeding 25% of the patient/family's annual income in a single year.

4) Employment status

If you are unemployed, you make less than 100% of FPL. Your medical bills are also going to be a significant portion of your income, because you have no income.

5) Uninsured

If you are uninsured, what is your uninsured or "self-pay" discount on charges? If you combine a standard 70% uninsured or "self-pay" discount with one of the previously mentioned poverty discounts and/or a catastrophic medical episode discounts, you will probably end up with a lower bill than a very well insured person.

Legal Implication of Financial Aid and Insured Patients

Let's suppose that you or the patient you represent has Medicare or any other type of insurance and you have clearly demonstrated that there is definite financial hardship in the form of poverty or medical catastrophe.

From time to time, you may have an uneducated biller or manager try to tell you that they cannot provide financial assistance to an insured patient because it is against the law. This is not true. There may be another motive, but this cannot be the "end all" reason.

For some time, U.S. hospitals did not offer financial assistance to Medicare beneficiaries that could not cover their cost-sharing liabilities (copays and deductibles) because they feared that the routine waiver of Medicare coinsurance and deductibles could violate a Federal law called the Anti-Kickback Statute[10].

In February of 2004, the secretary of the Department of Health and Human Services dispatched a letter to the American Hospital Association to dispel this myth[11]:

> *Your letter suggests that HHS regulations require hospitals to bill all patients using the same schedule of charges and suggests that as a result, the uninsured are forced to pay "full price" for their care. That suggestion is not correct and certainly does not accurately reflect my policy... the Office of Inspector General have prepared summaries of our policy that hospitals can use to assist the uninsured and underinsured.*
>
> *This guidance shows that hospitals can provide discounts to uninsured and underinsured patients who cannot afford their hospital bills and to Medicare beneficiaries who cannot afford*

10 Hospital Discounts Offered to Patients Who Cannot Afford to Pay Their Hospital Bills, Office of the Inspector General, February 2, 2004.
11 Letter from HHS Secretary Tommy Thompson to AHA President Richard Davidson, February 19, 2004.

their Medicare cost-sharing obligations. Nothing in the Medicare
program rules or regulations prohibit such discounts.

In fact, Medicare's fraud investigation unit, the Office of the Inspector General (OIG), has never brought a case against a hospital for discounting of bills for patients of limited means. The waiving of part or all of the Medicare cost liability of the patient may be acceptable for a "financially needy beneficiary" that can include "any reasonable measure of financial hardship."

The original law only meant to prohibit hospitals from using the Medicare coinsurance or deductible waivers exclusively to "drum up" new business. Basically, they cannot take out an ad in the paper that says "Seniors Welcome, We'll Waive Your Copays!" The only major stipulation is that hospitals may not use the waived copay or waived deductible as a write-off for bad debt.[12]

How to get out of collections

If your account was already sent to collections before you opened this book, please read the rest of this chapter first. You need to understand billers to do what I am about to explain. Let's review anyway.

1) Billers send accounts to collections *only* if they believe the patient is *able, but not willing* to pay. This means that they have given up hope on being able to collect the account themselves, yet they have no basis to waive any of the balance. They have no evidence that the patient is unable to pay, they just know that the patient has made little or no effort.

2) When this happens, they will classify the account as "bad debt." I will try not to be too technical, but when an account becomes bad debt, it changes from what accountants call an accounts receivable asset to a bad debt expense. They do this so they can clean up their accounts receivable books and so they can take advantage of the tax benefit of expensing the bad debt expense.

---

12 Unintended Consequences: How Federal Regulations and Hospital Policies Can Leave Patients in Debt, The Common Wealth Fund, June 2003.

3) When an account is sent to a collection agency, the patient normally only deals with the collectors. The biller is no longer involved.

Here is the trick. Collection agencies charge the provider to try to collect on the accounts. Normal fees are equal to 20%-30% of the balances collected. So if your delinquent account for $1,000 is sent to collection and the collector gets you to pay $500, the collector will keep $100-$150 and send the rest to the provider.

There are only two ways to get out of collections.

1) Pay down the balance you owe to the collector and live with the harassing calls, adverse effects to your credit score, and possible liens on your property until you do, or

2) You can seriously humble yourself to the biller and rationally convince them that they will make out as good or better if you pay them directly. This means you would have to come up with 70%-80% of what you owe. You are much less likely to get financial aid at this stage beyond matching the collection agency's 20%-30% collection charge, but you can get out of collections if you can convince the biller to reverse the "bad debt" adjustment and make your account active again.

I want to emphasize that #2 is very difficult. Let's say your chances of getting payment plans and financial aid within 30 days after the date of service are 90%. By comparison, if your account is sent to collections for no payments or bad communication for six months after the date of service I would estimate your chances of getting out of collections to be less than 30%. If your account is older than a year, I would estimate your chances at less than 10%. Though there is probably no financial aid to be had beyond matching the 70%-80% the collection agency would pay the provider, I would still go through the exercise of filling out the medical expense table in the previous chapter and doing the poverty and medical catastrophe calculations in this chapter. It certainly cannot hurt your chances.

OTHER ISSUES

There are a handful of other issues that you may encounter specific to elective surgery, escalating disputes to higher authorities, and unique situations with physicians as opposed to facilities.

Elective vs. non-elective care

You may get pushback on the financial aid front if your treatment was considered an "elective" service. Elective is a way of saying that you could have planned ahead to have the treatment done or that it was <u>not</u> done in an emergency situation. Conversely, non-elective means that you did not "elect" to have the treatment done because it was done in an emergency situation. A federal statute called EMTALA dictates that healthcare providers have to provide non-elective, emergency services, regardless of a patient's ability to pay. However, they can still legally refuse to perform elective procedures if there is evidence that payment will not occur.

I walk somewhat of a fine line here, because I am personally in the business of elective, outpatient surgery. This is a gray area anyway, so I'm going to do a bit of a philosophical analysis for you and then present my personal opinion.

I'm going to use the most common types of elective procedures as examples: cataract surgery, colonoscopies, and orthopedic joint arthroscopies.

Cataract surgery is a common elective procedure wherein an elderly individual has an artificial lens implanted in his or her eye, because the eye's natural lens has become cloudy and is impairing the ability to see clearly. Unfortunately, it can become expensive for the patient because they usually need to have both eyes done and the surgeon wants to do each several weeks apart. This is an example of a procedure that could be "put off" by the patient because it does not need to be done immediately. The patient is not in any physical pain. However, these are predominantly elderly people over 65 years old who may be severely restricted in their ability to drive and function independently without the ability to see. Yes, the procedure can be delayed and does not need to be done immediately, but it can be a considerable hardship to a person's lifestyle if it is put off too long

Colonoscopies are the most common elective procedure. They are done regularly after age 50 to screen for colon cancer and may be done at earlier ages if a patient has symptoms indicating there may be a problem. Screenings after age 50 are critical to diagnosing cancer before it advances too far. It is terrible to think that some people will not have the screening and perhaps let cancer advance because they can't or don't want to pay the $300 to $500 copay or deductible. Patients who have high deductibles may pay up to $1,000 for a colonoscopy.

Orthopedic arthroscopic surgery is similar in that it is a minimally invasive surgery that is important for diagnosing joint damage and tissue tears. Most of the corrective procedures can be done during the same surgery if a tissue tear is found. Again, "putting off" an arthroscopic surgery is possible, if the patient can live with the debilitating pain in his or her knees, hips, shoulders, or other joints.

You can probably see where I am going with this. "Elective" treatments are definitely necessary, and can be very painful and severely affect a person's lifestyle to decline treatment. Inevitably, the patient will need to have the elective procedure done.

I don't believe that patients who have elective medical procedures should not be eligible for financial aid; however, I also don't believe it is appropriate for patients to have an elective procedure done if they have no intention of paying their portion of the bill. If I were the financial aid "big cheese" at the American Hospital Association or the Ambulatory Surgery Center Association, I would make a policy that said:

Financial aid should be extended to patients who have elective procedures, as long as the patient applied for the financial aid and agreed to the terms before the procedure was performed. Financial aid may also be granted if some qualifying life event has occurred since the procedure was performed like loss of employment, change in insurance status, divorce, death of a spouse, and so on.

So, remembering that this a gray area where there really are no rules, it is my opinion that financial aid can and should be extended to patients who have elective procedures as long as the patient communicates hardship *prior* to service or if a qualifying life event has occurred to change the patient's circumstances since the procedure was performed.

Escalating

Only "escalate" issues to a higher authority if you absolutely have no alternative. When you "go over someone's head," you run a high risk of damaging your relationship with that person. You don't want to do this, because you probably will have to interact with the lower level person on a more regular basis. A prime example is telling a biller that you want to speak to his or her supervisor. You may or may not get the result you want, but the supervisor will still hand the phone back to the biller afterward.

If you do have to escalate, you want to do it calmly and rationally. You will feel more comfortable if you understand how billing departments are set up.

At a hospital, the billers probably work in a department called Patient Accounting, Patient Billing, or Patient Financial Services. Billers report to managers who report to Directors who report to VPs.

Hospital Escalation Chart

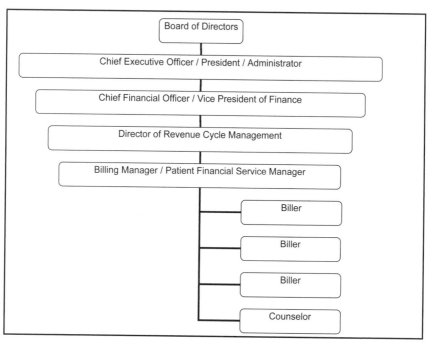

At a medium-size hospital like this one, you could theoretically escalate something five times from the biller all the way to the Board of Directors. In reality, I imagine you might be able to escalate something two desks from within the organization. That means Director of Revenue Cycle is probably as high as you will get.

I would say it is probably pretty unlikely you would get escalated to a VP or Chief Executive Officer. However, the community representatives on the Board of Directors are usually receptive if they are contacted directly. This is one thing I really like about community hospitals. The CEO's *real* boss is a group of normal people who live in the community or, possibly, business owners that run the local bank or hardware store. If you truly think the organization is not being fair or if you are in a very dire situation, the Board members are legitimate parties for an appeal.

A large physician group will look very similar to a hospital organization, except that the Board of Directors are replaced with "Physician Partners."

Smaller organizations like a small physician's office or an independent lab, imaging center, or surgery center will be much flatter. This applies if there is only one location. These types of businesses are lean on the staffing side, so you will probably deal with the same person every time. The office manager is probably empowered to be the main decision maker in this respect. I would estimate there is only a 20% chance you would ever speak to the Administrator and almost no chance you would ever speak to an owner.

Small Organization Escalation Chart

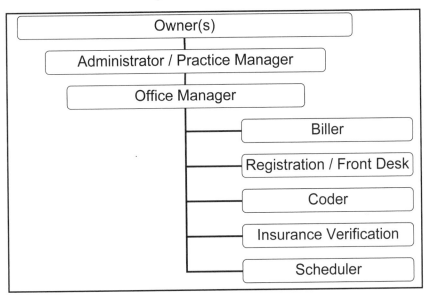

Balance billing

I'm sorry to say that there are physicians and other healthcare providers that engage in a sort of scam called "balance billing." Balance billing occurs when a healthcare provider bills a patient for some or the entire amount that should have been written off as the insurance discount (contractual allowance).

Whether it is truly balance billing will depend partially on whether the provider was in-network or out-of-network.

If the provider is in-network and billed you for more than the patient responsibility on your EOB, then this is a pretty "cut and dry" scam. Alert your insurance company and get a reference number on the call. The insurance company should have a billing specialist resolve this. In the event that you live in a state that has made "balance billing" illegal, I have letter templates for reporting in-network "balance billing" to your state's insurance commissioner and attorney general on this book's website at www.medicalbillsurvivalguide.com.

I have also posted the mail fraud report for the USPS mail inspection service on the website. Remember that a false "failure to pay" notice sent via the USPS is a federal mail fraud offense with criminal and civil penalties. Keep the envelope the bill came in!

If you saw an out-of-network (OON) provider, you may or may not be part of a scam. Here is how to tell:

Do you have out-of-network (OON) benefits?

1) Yes: If you do have an OON benefit, your OON deductible and coinsurance will apply first. The insurance company will pay the balance above and beyond your deductible and coinsurance just like normal. The only difference is that your OON deductible, copay, and coinsurance are probably more expensive than your in-network deductible, copay, and coinsurance.

2) No: If you don't have an OON benefit and saw this provider by accident, this is your responsibility. You need to tell them that you want to be treated like an uninsured or "self-pay" patient. They'll apply a standard discount for a patient without insurance to your balance.

If you have an OON benefit, did they "balance bill" you for more than your OON responsibility? If you have an OON benefit and the provider billed you for more than your OON deductible and coinsurance, you're probably caught in a scam. Here is what to do about it:

Check your EOB. Did insurance pay the provider? If your insurance did pay the provider, and the provider has billed you personally for more than your OON deductible and coinsurance, then they are definitely scamming you.

The reason providers always bill insurance, even if they are OON, is because some people have great OON coverage that pays 90% to 100% of full charges. Comparatively, this can be two or three times as much money as the provider receives for a normal patient. However, most people do not have great OON coverage. Providers "play the lottery" and still see OON patients because if one in ten OON claims does pay at this high rate, they pay so well that it more than makes up for the others.

This is often illegal and always wrong. Providers cannot "balance bill" just because they took a gamble and the insurance company's payment was too low. I have seen this quite a bit with small privately-owned for-profit healthcare businesses like physicians' offices, imaging centers, and surgery centers. Large not-for-profit hospitals and similar reputable organizations rarely engage in these nickel and dime types of practices.

Physicians

A physicians' ability to provide financial aid to patients is unique. I want you to understand why.

The plight of the American physician is really the same as the plight of the American small business owner. The small business owner strives to remain independent by warding off big business. They do not have the resources or the money to compete with their large competitors with regard to location, advertising, and highly paid employees. Therefore, they have to run faster, jump higher, and work much harder to maintain autonomy. If they can't keep up, they get swallowed up by a bigger company.

For the last seven years, Congress has voted not to reduce or increase Medicare payments to physicians. It is good for the physicians that payments have not been reduced, but unfortunate that they haven't been allowed any increases to cover inflation. Solo practice physicians have to give their staff members and office people raises every year and the cost of supplies and rent inevitably increases. If they don't receive payment increases to cover this, they have to see more and more patients to make up the difference. They have to work harder just to maintain.

Most facility-based providers like hospitals, surgery centers, and imaging centers have experienced reimbursement fluctuations from year to year. They generally receive inflationary increases, but also receive reductions, as payment systems are periodically updated to become more equitable to the various types of providers. Medicare is a "budget-neutral" program. This means that when money is reduced in one area, it has to be spent in another area within Medicare. Here are examples for four different types of healthcare providers:

1) Hospital reimbursement is updated often to better reward hospitals that provide higher quality service and disincentivize hospitals that do not measure up. The overall effect is neutral. Medicare just moves money around to encourage better care.

2) Ambulatory surgery centers have recently received payment cuts to the most common types of procedures like colonoscopies and cataract surgeries, while less common orthopedic and urology procedures are paid at higher rates. This encourages the most common procedures to be done at specialty centers in a sort of efficient "factory style."

3) Imaging centers also received a big cut in reimbursement for MRIs and CAT scans several years ago when a law called the Deficient Reduction Act (DRA) went into effect. This made it very difficult to compete and many providers went out of business or were bought by bigger companies.

4) Home healthcare Medicare reimbursement was totally changed back in the year 2000. The new system rewarded efficient home health agencies and penalized inefficient home health agencies. The number of providers reduced from 10,000 to 7,000 within a few years.

The overall effect I'm trying to demonstrate is consolidation. Generally speaking, when the market becomes more and more competitive, weaker businesses will either fail or sell out to bigger, stronger businesses. This is the same in healthcare.

Even hospitals and regional health systems have merged into giant "mega health systems" as things have become more difficult. Prime examples are the four Catholic "mega systems." Each one represents multiple regional health systems and individual hospitals that banned together.

- Catholic Healthcare West (CHW) 40 hospitals plus affiliates
- Catholic Healthcare East (CHE) 40 hospitals plus affiliates
- Catholic Health Partners (CHP) 38 hospitals plus affiliates
- Catholic Health Initiatives (CHI) 75 hospitals plus affiliates

I want you to understand this effect because it is happening to physicians too. The larger physician groups that are pooling their resources are going to be in a better position to offer financial assistance than the "one-off" physicians who have to work much harder and see many more patients just to get by.

Here is a test to see if your physician is overworked. If you consistently have to wait over 45 minutes after your appointment time to see your physician, they are "overbooking" or "double booking" because they want to squeeze in as many patients as they can in a limited amount of time.

In the last few years, we have seen more physicians become "employees" of hospitals or "salaried partners" of larger medical groups because it is too difficult to have a solo practice. This is good for patients that are experiencing financial hardship, because these physician practices operate more like professional organizations with formalized policies and rules than a smaller self-proprietorship where one person is the authority for every decision.

This is not a rule and I am not condemning solo practitioners in any way. My own primary care physician is a solo practitioner. Many solo practitioners have very well-run offices and will have no problem providing care for patients of limited means.

However, do not despair if you are refused service by a physician for reasons of uninsured status or inability to meet high deductibles. There are 600,000 physicians in the U.S. It will not be difficult to find someone else to care for you.

OTHER RESOURCES

There are four other resources available to you.

Online Insurance Portal

If you have insurance, your insurance company provides you with excellent resources including online access to claims, EOBs, your benefit plan, their in-network provider list, and probably pricing tools that will tell you what your patient responsibilities will be for different types of care at different facilities. I have put the websites for the five largest U.S. insurance carriers below. You may have to register if you have not signed on before.

1. United Healthcare: www.myuhc.com

2. Wellpoint Anthem: www.anthem.com

3. Aetna: www.aetna.com

4. Humana: www.humana.com

5. Cigna: my.cigna.com

Patient financing companies

Beware of revolving credit. Just like credit cards, this can be a good thing if you have the discipline to make your payments on time and have the whole amount paid off by the end of your term. The most popular service that I'm aware of is Care Credit. Over 100,000 medical providers now accept Care Credit.

Care Credit operates the same way as a Home Depot card. It is an "interest free" credit card as long as you make the minimum monthly payment, and pay off the whole amount within the allotted payment plan. The *catch* is that if you make the minimum monthly payments, you won't have the whole amount paid off within the allotted payment plan.

For example, let's say you pay for your $1,000 surgery deductible with Care Credit on a 12 month plan. You make your minimum monthly payment every month of $55. However, at month 12, you get your last statement and the balance is $490. You have to make a balloon payment to pay off the balance, or they will back-date the interest on the whole balance at a pretty high interest rate.

Providers love Care Credit because it pays them upfront just like a credit card, and they can close your account. The provider doesn't have to call you every month, doesn't have to send you statements, and doesn't have to send anybody to collections.

The Foundation for Health Coverage Education

The chapter entitled "Things to know if you don't have insurance" described the four largest public insurance programs in the U.S. These are Medicare, Medicaid, SCHIP, and COBRA.

However, each state in the U.S. has unique public insurance programs that others may not. The Foundation for Health Coverage Education has assembled a very useful matrix that identifies the unique eligibility requirements, costs, benefits, and contact information for eight programs in each state. FHCE also has a 24-hour hotline with consultants that will help you find programs for which you are eligible. This matrix is an excellent free resource that can be downloaded at www.coverageforall.org.

I have attached a similar, but smaller matrix in the appendix that includes eligibility criteria for Medicaid and SCHIP in each state.

The author's website and community forum

I believe the items I have highlighted in this book are the most common problems that normal people experience with overwhelming medical costs. It is far from a comprehensive guide to every medical bill problem that exists.

If executed correctly, I expect these strategies will improve the situation of nine out of ten people who need help with their medical bills.

If you have difficulty understanding something I've discussed here or more importantly, if you have difficulty communicating something I've discussed here to a biller, I invite you to post a request for assistance on our free community forum at www.medicalbillsurvivalguide.com. The forum creates a venue for people whom have experienced similar problems to share their stories. I look forward to hearing from you and, I hope, to helping you with your bills.

APPENDIX

The Appendix contains Medicaid and SCHIP eligibility information for every state and the Distrtict of Columbia.

While 100% of FPL is the minimum Medicaid eligibility level set by the federal government for children 6-19 years old, the two healthcare reform bills currently being considered in early 2010 would raise minimum coverage to 150% of FPL (HR 3962) or 133% of FPL (HR 3590) in states that have adopted the minimum Medicaid eligibility level.

Please do not dismiss your eligibility for these programs easily. The eligibility levels change annually, many states are offering subsidized "buy-in" options, and this reference will quickly become outdated. I have included web addresses and phone numbers for each program so that you can contact your state directly for the most current information.

Alabama

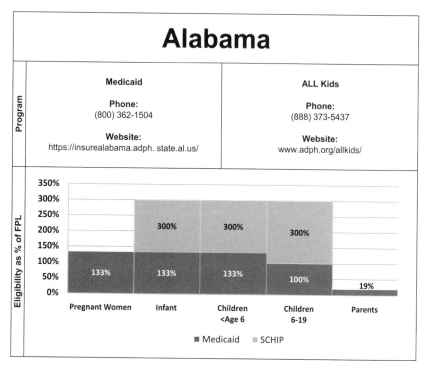

	Medicaid	ALL Kids
Program	**Medicaid** Phone: (800) 362-1504 Website: https://insurealabama.adph. state.al.us/	**ALL Kids** Phone: (888) 373-5437 Website: www.adph.org/allkids/

Eligibility as % of FPL

Pregnant Women	Infant	Children <Age 6	Children 6-19	Parents
133%	133% / 300%	133% / 300%	100% / 300%	19%

■ Medicaid ■ SCHIP

Alaska

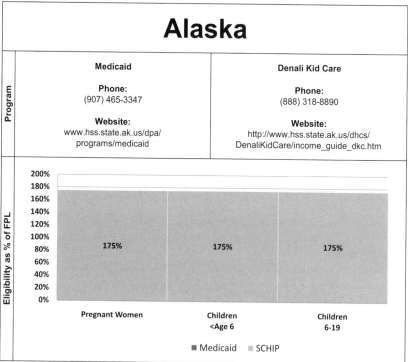

	Medicaid	Denali Kid Care
Program	**Medicaid** Phone: (907) 465-3347 Website: www.hss.state.ak.us/dpa/ programs/medicaid	**Denali Kid Care** Phone: (888) 318-8890 Website: http://www.hss.state.ak.us/dhcs/ DenaliKidCare/income_guide_dkc.htm

Eligibility as % of FPL

Pregnant Women	Children <Age 6	Children 6-19
175%	175%	175%

■ Medicaid ■ SCHIP

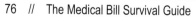

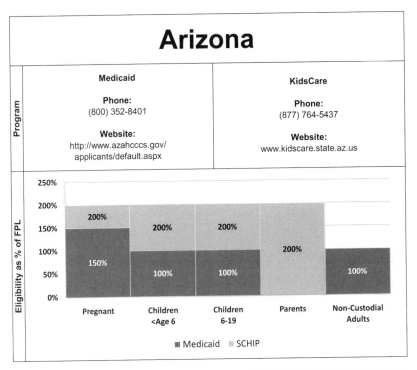

Arizona

Medicaid	KidsCare
Phone: (800) 352-8401	**Phone:** (877) 764-5437
Website: http://www.azahcccs.gov/ applicants/default.aspx	**Website:** www.kidscare.state.az.us

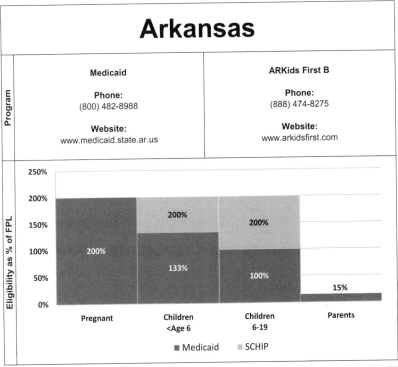

Arkansas

Medicaid	ARKids First B
Phone: (800) 482-8988	**Phone:** (888) 474-8275
Website: www.medicaid.state.ar.us	**Website:** www.arkidsfirst.com

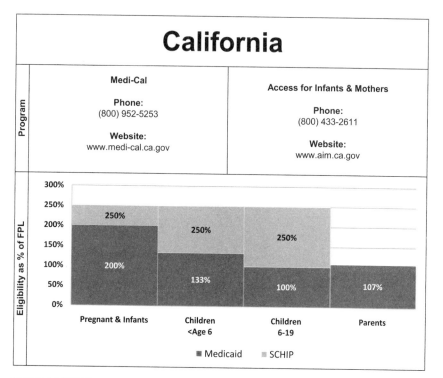

California

Medi-Cal	Access for Infants & Mothers
Phone: (800) 952-5253	Phone: (800) 433-2611
Website: www.medi-cal.ca.gov	Website: www.aim.ca.gov

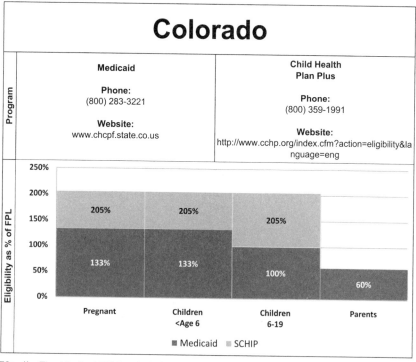

Colorado

Medicaid	Child Health Plan Plus
Phone: (800) 283-3221	Phone: (800) 359-1991
Website: www.chcpf.state.co.us	Website: http://www.cchp.org/index.cfm?action=eligibility&language=eng

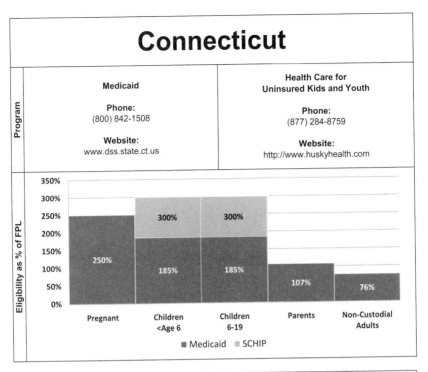

Connecticut

Medicaid	Health Care for Uninsured Kids and Youth
Phone: (800) 842-1508	**Phone:** (877) 284-8759
Website: www.dss.state.ct.us	**Website:** http://www.huskyhealth.com

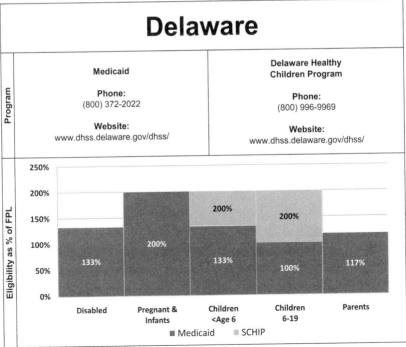

Delaware

Medicaid	Delaware Healthy Children Program
Phone: (800) 372-2022	**Phone:** (800) 996-9969
Website: www.dhss.delaware.gov/dhss/	**Website:** www.dhss.delaware.gov/dhss/

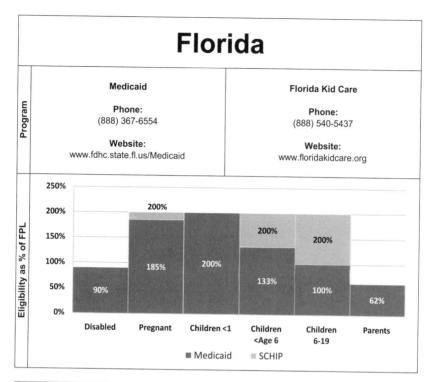

Florida

Medicaid	Florida Kid Care
Phone: (888) 367-6554	Phone: (888) 540-5437
Website: www.fdhc.state.fl.us/Medicaid	Website: www.floridakidcare.org

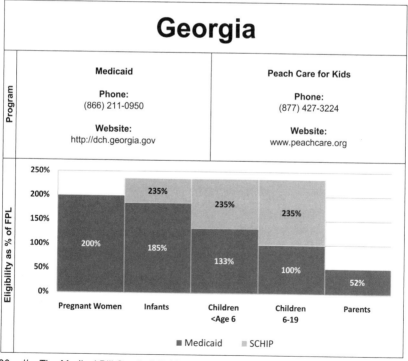

Georgia

Medicaid	Peach Care for Kids
Phone: (866) 211-0950	Phone: (877) 427-3224
Website: http://dch.georgia.gov	Website: www.peachcare.org

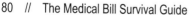

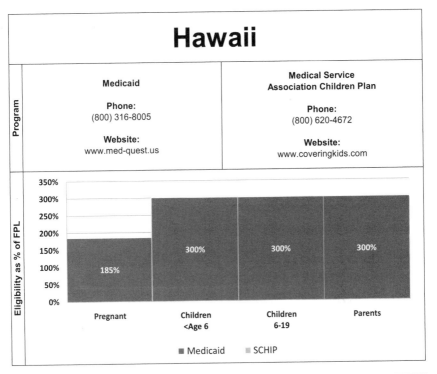

Hawaii

Program	Medicaid Phone: (800) 316-8005 Website: www.med-quest.us	Medical Service Association Children Plan Phone: (800) 620-4672 Website: www.coveringkids.com

Eligibility as % of FPL

- Pregnant: 185% (Medicaid)
- Children <Age 6: 300%
- Children 6-19: 300%
- Parents: 300%

■ Medicaid ■ SCHIP

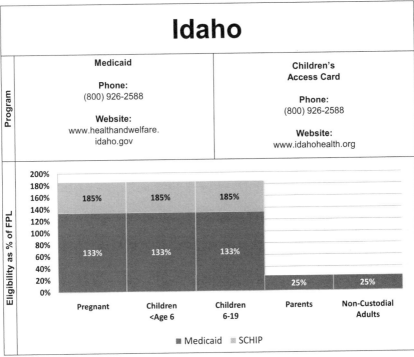

Idaho

Program	Medicaid Phone: (800) 926-2588 Website: www.healthandwelfare. idaho.gov	Children's Access Card Phone: (800) 926-2588 Website: www.idahohealth.org

Eligibility as % of FPL

- Pregnant: 133% (Medicaid), 185% (SCHIP)
- Children <Age 6: 133% (Medicaid), 185% (SCHIP)
- Children 6-19: 133% (Medicaid), 185% (SCHIP)
- Parents: 25%
- Non-Custodial Adults: 25%

■ Medicaid ■ SCHIP

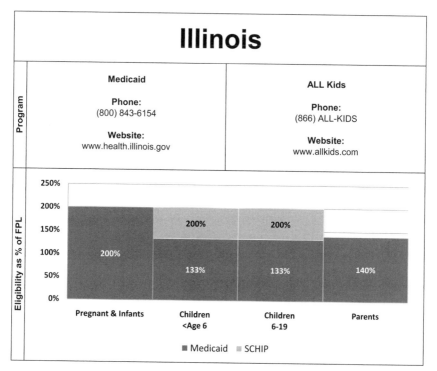

Illinois

Medicaid	ALL Kids
Phone: (800) 843-6154	Phone: (866) ALL-KIDS
Website: www.health.illinois.gov	Website: www.allkids.com

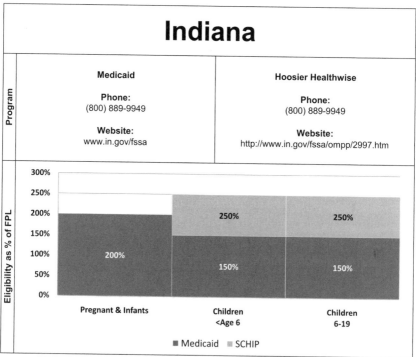

Indiana

Medicaid	Hoosier Healthwise
Phone: (800) 889-9949	Phone: (800) 889-9949
Website: www.in.gov/fssa	Website: http://www.in.gov/fssa/ompp/2997.htm

Iowa

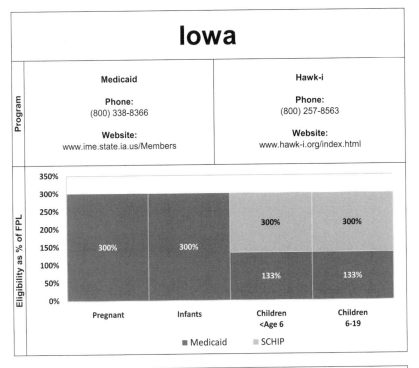

Program	Medicaid	Hawk-i
	Medicaid Phone: (800) 338-8366 Website: www.ime.state.ia.us/Members	**Hawk-i** Phone: (800) 257-8563 Website: www.hawk-i.org/index.html

Kansas

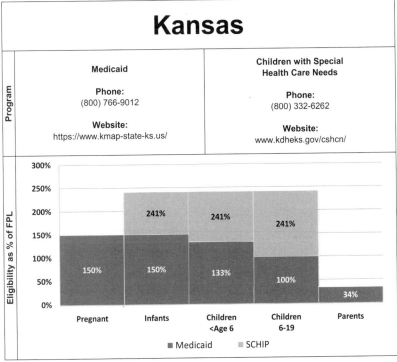

Program	Medicaid	Children with Special Health Care Needs
	Medicaid Phone: (800) 766-9012 Website: https://www.kmap-state-ks.us/	**Children with Special Health Care Needs** Phone: (800) 332-6262 Website: www.kdheks.gov/cshcn/

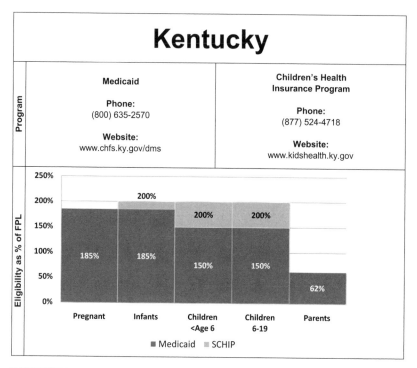

Kentucky

Medicaid	Children's Health Insurance Program
Phone: (800) 635-2570	**Phone:** (877) 524-4718
Website: www.chfs.ky.gov/dms	**Website:** www.kidshealth.ky.gov

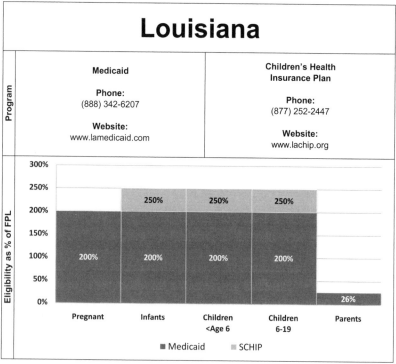

Louisiana

Medicaid	Children's Health Insurance Plan
Phone: (888) 342-6207	**Phone:** (877) 252-2447
Website: www.lamedicaid.com	**Website:** www.lachip.org

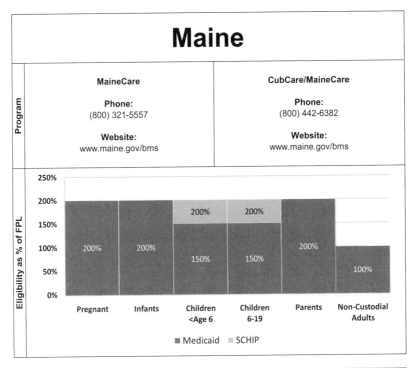

Maine

MaineCare	CubCare/MaineCare
Phone: (800) 321-5557	Phone: (800) 442-6382
Website: www.maine.gov/bms	Website: www.maine.gov/bms

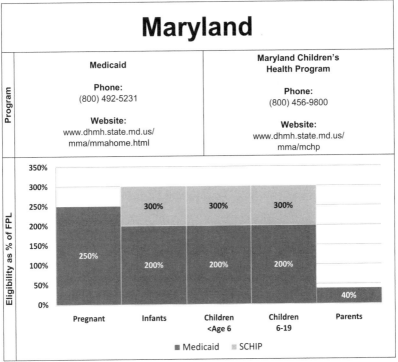

Maryland

Medicaid	Maryland Children's Health Program
Phone: (800) 492-5231	Phone: (800) 456-9800
Website: www.dhmh.state.md.us/ mma/mmahome.html	Website: www.dhmh.state.md.us/ mma/mchp

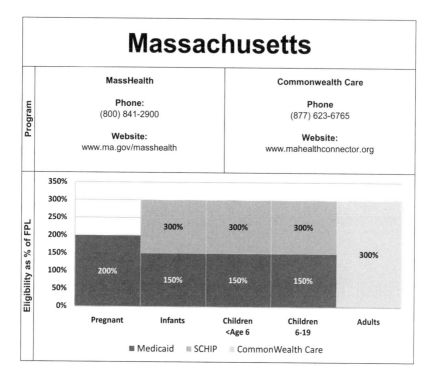

Massachusetts

MassHealth	Commonwealth Care
Phone: (800) 841-2900	Phone (877) 623-6765
Website: www.ma.gov/masshealth	Website: www.mahealthconnector.org

Eligibility as % of FPL

- Pregnant: 200%
- Infants: 150% / 300%
- Children <Age 6: 150% / 300%
- Children 6-19: 150% / 300%
- Adults: 300%

■ Medicaid ■ SCHIP ■ CommonWealth Care

Note: Massachusetts is the frontrunner state on healthcare reform. It was the first state to create a health insurance mandate requiring all resident to acquire health insurance. This is accomplished through a combination of free programs and sliding scale discounts for the poor as well as tax penalties on those that voluntarily choose not to purchase health insurance. The mandate is facilitated by the Commonwealth Health Insurance Authority.

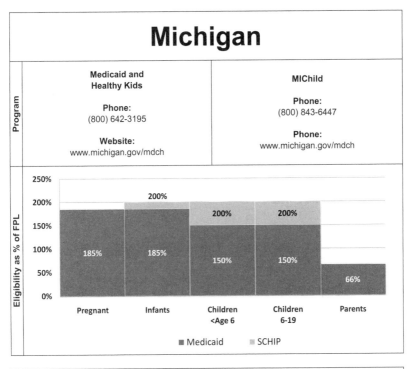

Michigan

Medicaid and Healthy Kids	MIChild
Phone: (800) 642-3195	Phone: (800) 843-6447
Website: www.michigan.gov/mdch	Phone: www.michigan.gov/mdch

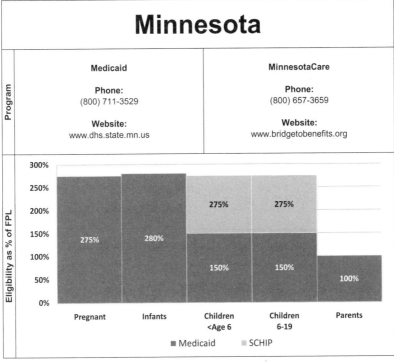

Minnesota

Medicaid	MinnesotaCare
Phone: (800) 711-3529	Phone: (800) 657-3659
Website: www.dhs.state.mn.us	Website: www.bridgetobenefits.org

Mississippi

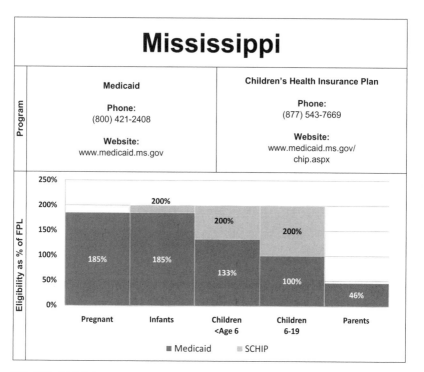

Program	Medicaid	Children's Health Insurance Plan
	Phone: (800) 421-2408	**Phone:** (877) 543-7669
	Website: www.medicaid.ms.gov	**Website:** www.medicaid.ms.gov/ chip.aspx

Missouri

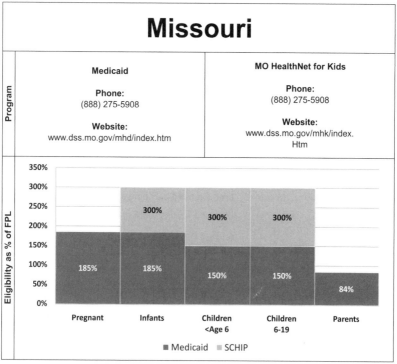

Program	Medicaid	MO HealthNet for Kids
	Phone: (888) 275-5908	**Phone:** (888) 275-5908
	Website: www.dss.mo.gov/mhd/index.htm	**Website:** www.dss.mo.gov/mhk/index. Htm

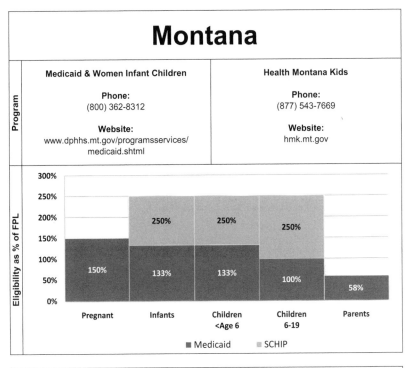

Montana

Medicaid & Women Infant Children	Health Montana Kids
Phone: (800) 362-8312	**Phone:** (877) 543-7669
Website: www.dphhs.mt.gov/programsservices/ medicaid.shtml	**Website:** hmk.mt.gov

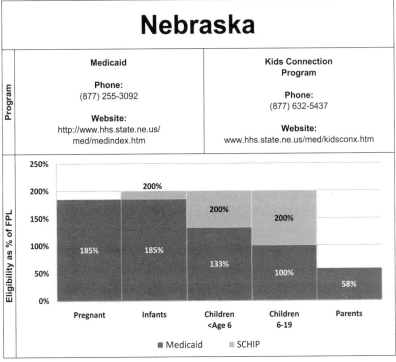

Nebraska

Medicaid	Kids Connection Program
Phone: (877) 255-3092	**Phone:** (877) 632-5437
Website: http://www.hhs.state.ne.us/ med/medindex.htm	**Website:** www.hhs.state.ne.us/med/kidsconx.htm

Nevada

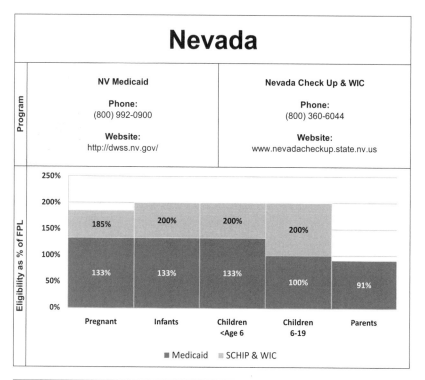

	NV Medicaid	Nevada Check Up & WIC
Program	**Phone:** (800) 992-0900 **Website:** http://dwss.nv.gov/	**Phone:** (800) 360-6044 **Website:** www.nevadacheckup.state.nv.us

Eligibility as % of FPL

	Pregnant	Infants	Children <Age 6	Children 6-19	Parents
SCHIP & WIC	185%	200%	200%	200%	
Medicaid	133%	133%	133%	100%	91%

■ Medicaid   ■ SCHIP & WIC

New Hampshire

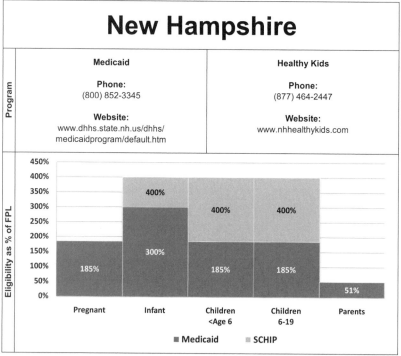

	Medicaid	Healthy Kids
Program	**Phone:** (800) 852-3345 **Website:** www.dhhs.state.nh.us/dhhs/ medicaidprogram/default.htm	**Phone:** (877) 464-2447 **Website:** www.nhhealthykids.com

Eligibility as % of FPL

	Pregnant	Infant	Children <Age 6	Children 6-19	Parents
SCHIP		400%	400%	400%	
Medicaid	185%	300%	185%	185%	51%

■ Medicaid   ■ SCHIP

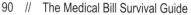

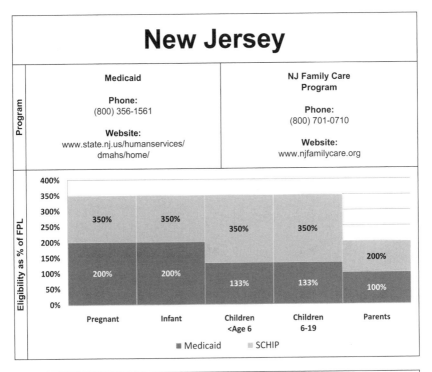

New Jersey

	Medicaid	NJ Family Care Program
Program	Phone: (800) 356-1561	Phone: (800) 701-0710
	Website: www.state.nj.us/humanservices/dmahs/home/	Website: www.njfamilycare.org

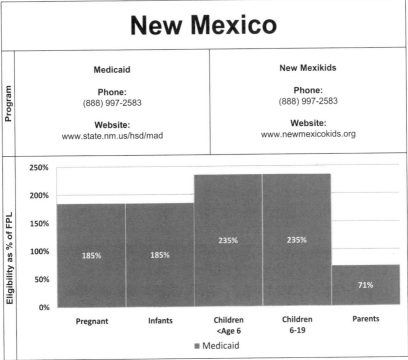

New Mexico

	Medicaid	New Mexikids
Program	Phone: (888) 997-2583	Phone: (888) 997-2583
	Website: www.state.nm.us/hsd/mad	Website: www.newmexicokids.org

New York

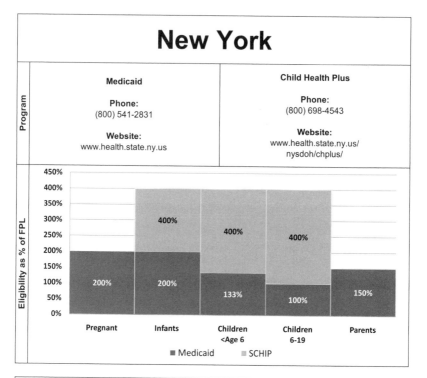

Medicaid	**Child Health Plus**
Phone: (800) 541-2831	**Phone:** (800) 698-4543
Website: www.health.state.ny.us	**Website:** www.health.state.ny.us/ nysdoh/chplus/

Program / Eligibility as % of FPL

- Pregnant: 200%
- Infants: 200% / 400%
- Children <Age 6: 133% / 400%
- Children 6-19: 100% / 400%
- Parents: 150%

■ Medicaid ■ SCHIP

North Carolina

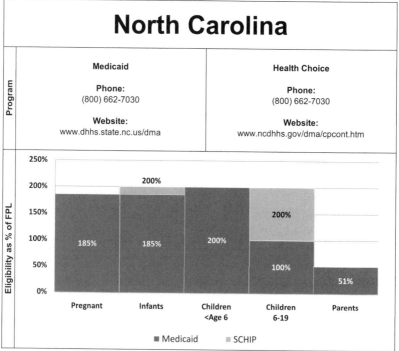

Medicaid	**Health Choice**
Phone: (800) 662-7030	**Phone:** (800) 662-7030
Website: www.dhhs.state.nc.us/dma	**Website:** www.ncdhhs.gov/dma/cpcont.htm

Program / Eligibility as % of FPL

- Pregnant: 185%
- Infants: 185% / 200%
- Children <Age 6: 200%
- Children 6-19: 100% / 200%
- Parents: 51%

■ Medicaid ■ SCHIP

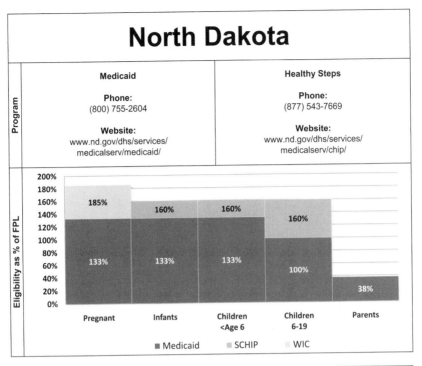

North Dakota

Medicaid	Healthy Steps
Phone: (800) 755-2604	Phone: (877) 543-7669
Website: www.nd.gov/dhs/services/ medicalserv/medicaid/	Website: www.nd.gov/dhs/services/ medicalserv/chip/

Eligibility as % of FPL

- Pregnant: 185% / 133%
- Infants: 160% / 133%
- Children <Age 6: 160% / 133%
- Children 6-19: 160% / 100%
- Parents: 38%

■ Medicaid ■ SCHIP ■ WIC

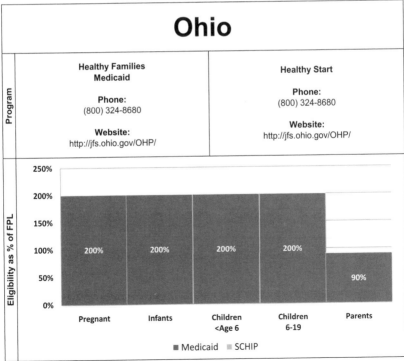

Ohio

Healthy Families Medicaid	Healthy Start
Phone: (800) 324-8680	Phone: (800) 324-8680
Website: http://jfs.ohio.gov/OHP/	Website: http://jfs.ohio.gov/OHP/

Eligibility as % of FPL

- Pregnant: 200%
- Infants: 200%
- Children <Age 6: 200%
- Children 6-19: 200%
- Parents: 90%

■ Medicaid ■ SCHIP

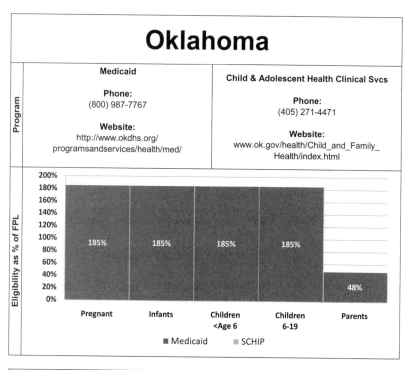

Oklahoma

Medicaid	Child & Adolescent Health Clinical Svcs
Phone: (800) 987-7767	**Phone:** (405) 271-4471
Website: http://www.okdhs.org/ programsandservices/health/med/	**Website:** www.ok.gov/health/Child_and_Family_ Health/index.html

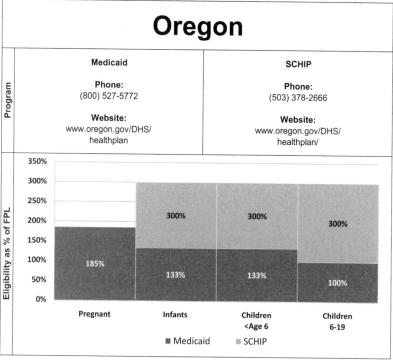

Oregon

Medicaid	SCHIP
Phone: (800) 527-5772	**Phone:** (503) 378-2666
Website: www.oregon.gov/DHS/ healthplan	**Website:** www.oregon.gov/DHS/ healthplan/

Pennsylvania

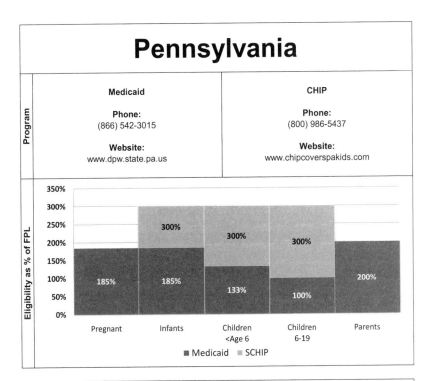

	Medicaid	CHIP
Program	Phone: (866) 542-3015 Website: www.dpw.state.pa.us	Phone: (800) 986-5437 Website: www.chipcoverspakids.com

Eligibility as % of FPL

- Pregnant: 185% (Medicaid)
- Infants: 185% (Medicaid), 300% (SCHIP)
- Children <Age 6: 133% (Medicaid), 300% (SCHIP)
- Children 6-19: 100% (Medicaid), 300% (SCHIP)
- Parents: 200% (Medicaid)

■ Medicaid ■ SCHIP

Rhode Island

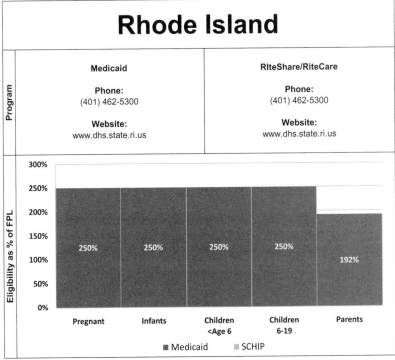

	Medicaid	RIteShare/RiteCare
Program	Phone: (401) 462-5300 Website: www.dhs.state.ri.us	Phone: (401) 462-5300 Website: www.dhs.state.ri.us

Eligibility as % of FPL

- Pregnant: 250%
- Infants: 250%
- Children <Age 6: 250%
- Children 6-19: 250%
- Parents: 192%

■ Medicaid ■ SCHIP

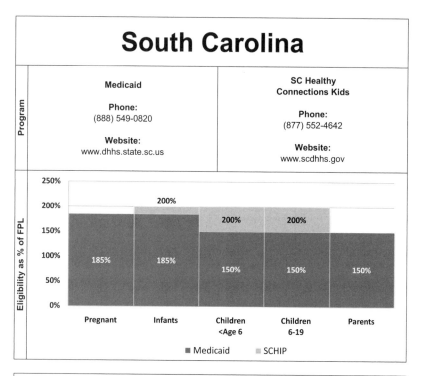

South Carolina

Program	Medicaid Phone: (888) 549-0820 Website: www.dhhs.state.sc.us	SC Healthy Connections Kids Phone: (877) 552-4642 Website: www.scdhhs.gov

Eligibility as % of FPL

	Pregnant	Infants	Children <Age 6	Children 6-19	Parents
Medicaid	185%	185%	150%	150%	150%
SCHIP		200%	200%	200%	

■ Medicaid ■ SCHIP

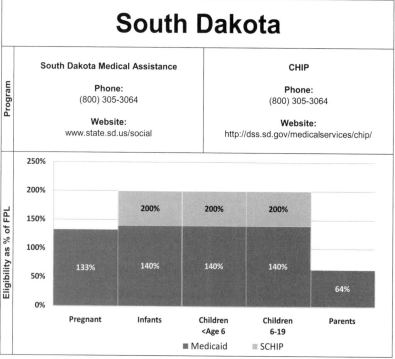

South Dakota

Program	South Dakota Medical Assistance Phone: (800) 305-3064 Website: www.state.sd.us/social	CHIP Phone: (800) 305-3064 Website: http://dss.sd.gov/medicalservices/chip/

Eligibility as % of FPL

	Pregnant	Infants	Children <Age 6	Children 6-19	Parents
Medicaid	133%	140%	140%	140%	64%
SCHIP		200%	200%	200%	

■ Medicaid ■ SCHIP

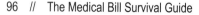

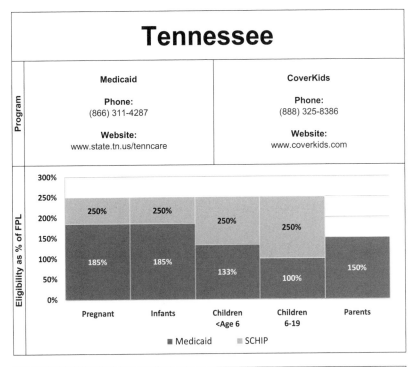

Tennessee

Medicaid	CoverKids
Phone: (866) 311-4287	Phone: (888) 325-8386
Website: www.state.tn.us/tenncare	Website: www.coverkids.com

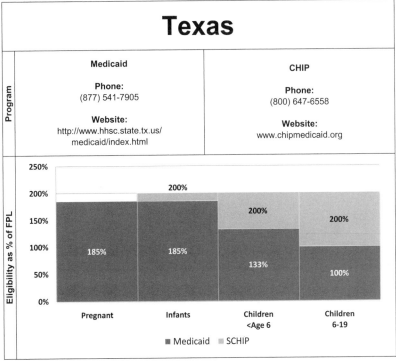

Texas

Medicaid	CHIP
Phone: (877) 541-7905	Phone: (800) 647-6558
Website: http://www.hhsc.state.tx.us/medicaid/index.html	Website: www.chipmedicaid.org

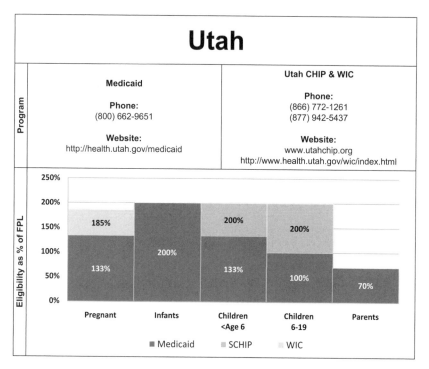

Utah

Medicaid	Utah CHIP & WIC
Phone: (800) 662-9651	**Phone:** (866) 772-1261 (877) 942-5437
Website: http://health.utah.gov/medicaid	**Website:** www.utahchip.org http://www.health.utah.gov/wic/index.html

Eligibility as % of FPL

Pregnant	Infants	Children <Age 6	Children 6-19	Parents
185% / 133%	200%	200% / 133%	200% / 100%	70%

■ Medicaid ■ SCHIP ■ WIC

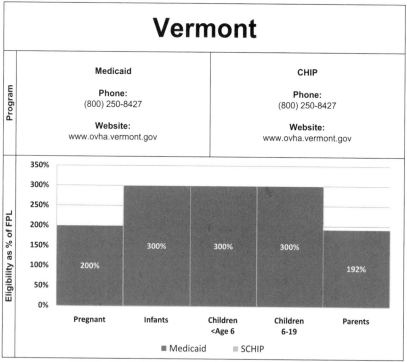

Vermont

Medicaid	CHIP
Phone: (800) 250-8427	**Phone:** (800) 250-8427
Website: www.ovha.vermont.gov	**Website:** www.ovha.vermont.gov

Eligibility as % of FPL

Pregnant	Infants	Children <Age 6	Children 6-19	Parents
200%	300%	300%	300%	192%

■ Medicaid ■ SCHIP

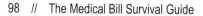

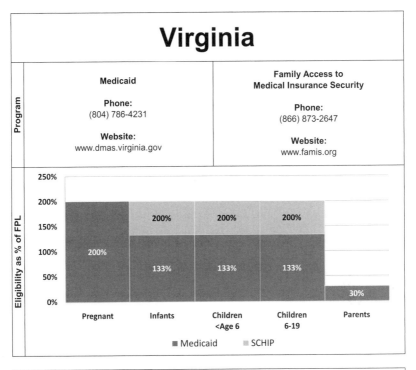

Virginia

Medicaid	Family Access to Medical Insurance Security
Phone: (804) 786-4231	**Phone:** (866) 873-2647
Website: www.dmas.virginia.gov	**Website:** www.famis.org

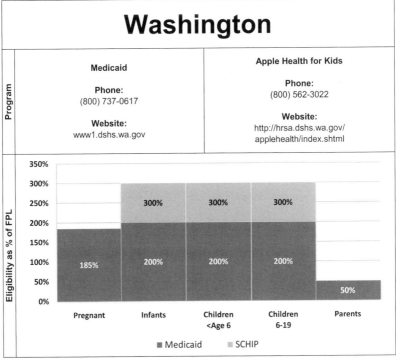

Washington

Medicaid	Apple Health for Kids
Phone: (800) 737-0617	**Phone:** (800) 562-3022
Website: www1.dshs.wa.gov	**Website:** http://hrsa.dshs.wa.gov/applehealth/index.shtml

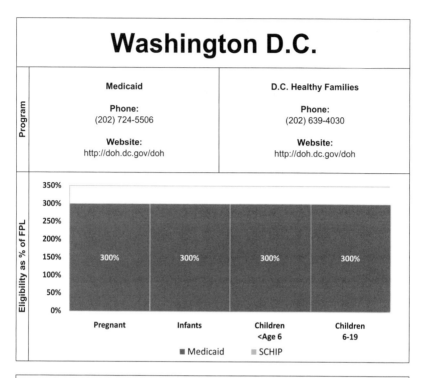

Washington D.C.

Medicaid	D.C. Healthy Families
Phone: (202) 724-5506	**Phone:** (202) 639-4030
Website: http://doh.dc.gov/doh	**Website:** http://doh.dc.gov/doh

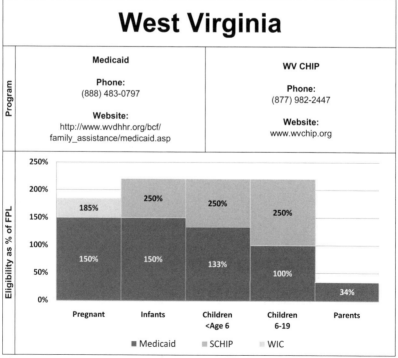

West Virginia

Medicaid	WV CHIP
Phone: (888) 483-0797	**Phone:** (877) 982-2447
Website: http://www.wvdhhr.org/bcf/ family_assistance/medicaid.asp	**Website:** www.wvchip.org

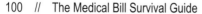